Power Yoga

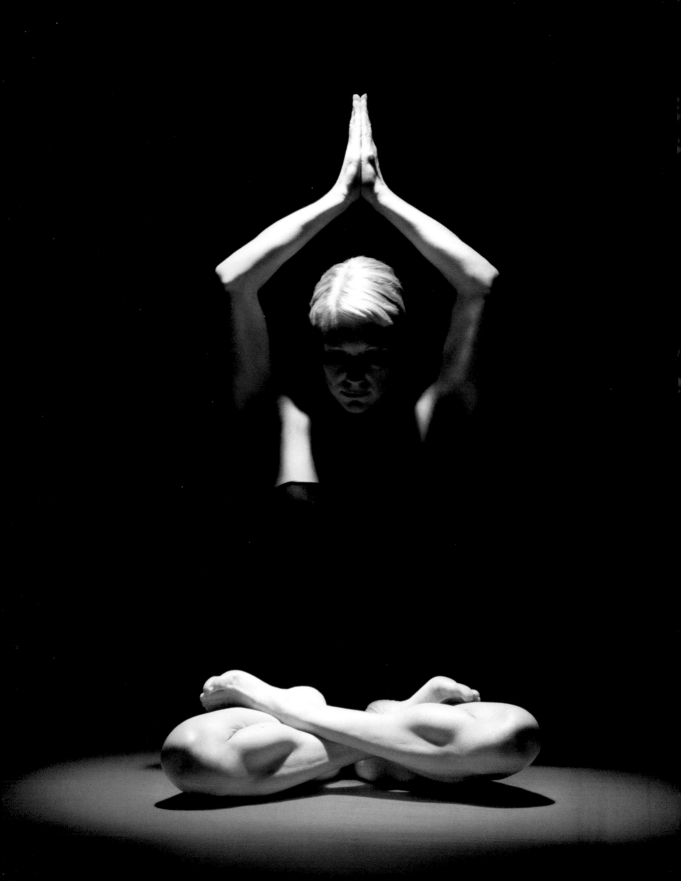

Ulrica Norberg   Photos: Andreas Lundberg

Power Yoga

An Individualized Approach to Strength, Grace, and Inner Peace

Translated by Dorthe Nors

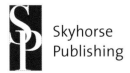

Skyhorse
Publishing

www.skyhorsepublishing.com

ISBN: 1-60239-037-1
978-1-60239-037-9

10 9 8 7 6 5 4 3 2 1

Library of Congress Cataloging-in-Publication Data
Norberg, Ulrica.
    Power yoga : an individualized approach to strength,
    grace, and inner peace / by Ulrica Norberg ; photos,
    Andreas Lundberg ; translated by Dorthe Nors.
        p.   cm.
    Includes bibliographical references and index.
    ISBN-13: 978-1-60239-037-9
    ISBN-10: 1-60239-037-1
    1. Yoga.   I. Title.

  RA781.7.N668   2007
  613.7'046—dc22   2006038124

Printed in China

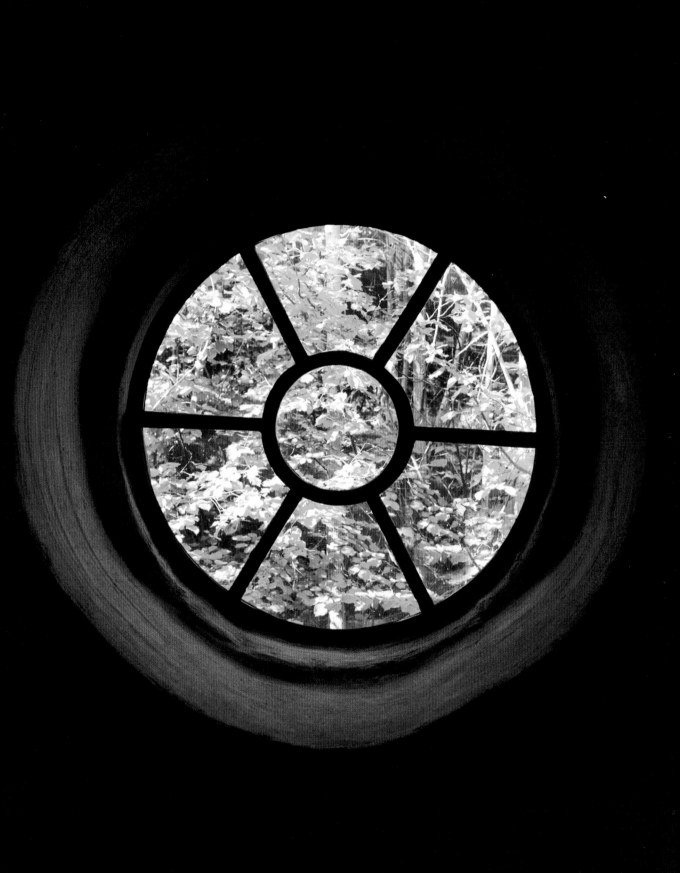

Publisher's Note:

Before following any advice or practice suggested in this book, it is recommended that you consult your doctor as to its suitability, especially if you suffer from any health problems or special conditions. The publishers, the author, and the photographers cannot accept responsibility for any injuries or damage incurred as a result of following the exercises in this book, or of using the therapeutic methods described or mentioned here.

Contents

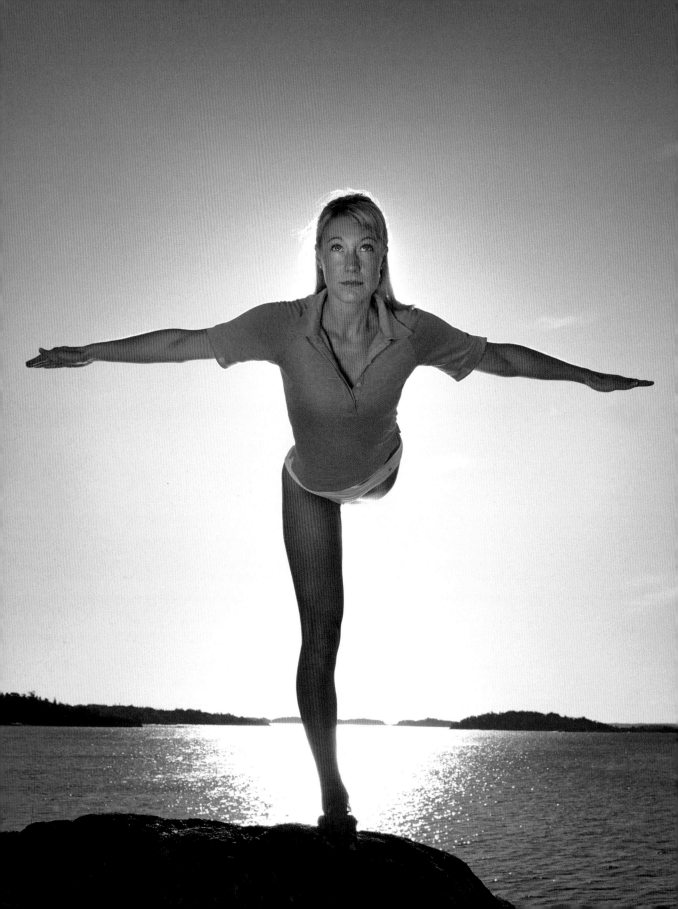

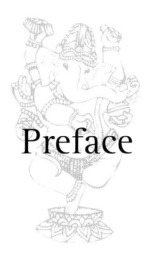

Preface

Einstein taught us that the physical body just like all material objects is an illusion and an attempt to handle it can be like grasping at a shadow and missing out on the substance. The unseen world is the real world and when we are willing to explore the unseen levels of our bodies we can gain access to the immensely creative power that is placed within our source.[1] *— Deepak Chopra*

This book introduces the basic ideas, movements, and techniques in the dynamic Hatha Yoga style called *Power Yoga*. If this is your first introduction to yoga, it is important to take one step and one day at a time. Try to think of yoga as learning an alphabet; you move from letter to letter but never jump directly from to A to Z. Each letter is unique and important in building language. It is my hope that this book can shed light on yoga in an attainable way and give you insight into its philosophy and structure.

Some people who practice yoga see it entirely as a physical way of training that offers flexibility, strength, endurance, and balance. Others see yoga as a spiritual and mental path to knowledge and deeper understanding. Neither path is right or wrong. You are your own master. Yoga offers a long list of positive effects, and if you train regularly, you will feel a growing positive difference—not only in your body, but also mentally and spiritually.

Whatever your intent, Power Yoga can teach you to become stronger, produce positive results, and help you feel better!

It is important that you listen to your body when you do the exercises. If it's possible, aim for a feeling of comfort in every pose, but also challenge your body. Most importantly, follow the rhythm of the breath. This book is not meant to be a substitute for an experienced yoga teacher who can guide you in your training and evaluate your qualifications, needs, and development, but it is my hope that this book can offer an exciting introduction to yoga. The first three chapters describe the philosophical ideas behind yoga training. The next three chapters contain yoga exercises that circle around Sun Salutation-sequences, followed by standing and seated poses. After this follows a chapter on physical and mental relaxation, and at the end of the book, you'll find some of the most frequently asked questions and answers about yoga.

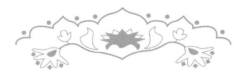

Health is the greatest prize, contentment is the mightiest wealth. A reliable friend is the best kinsman and Nirvana[2] is the ultimate happiness. —Buddha

[1] *Ageless Body, Timeless Mind—see bibliography.*
[2] *Nirvana = state of completeness in which the soul is united with the universe.*

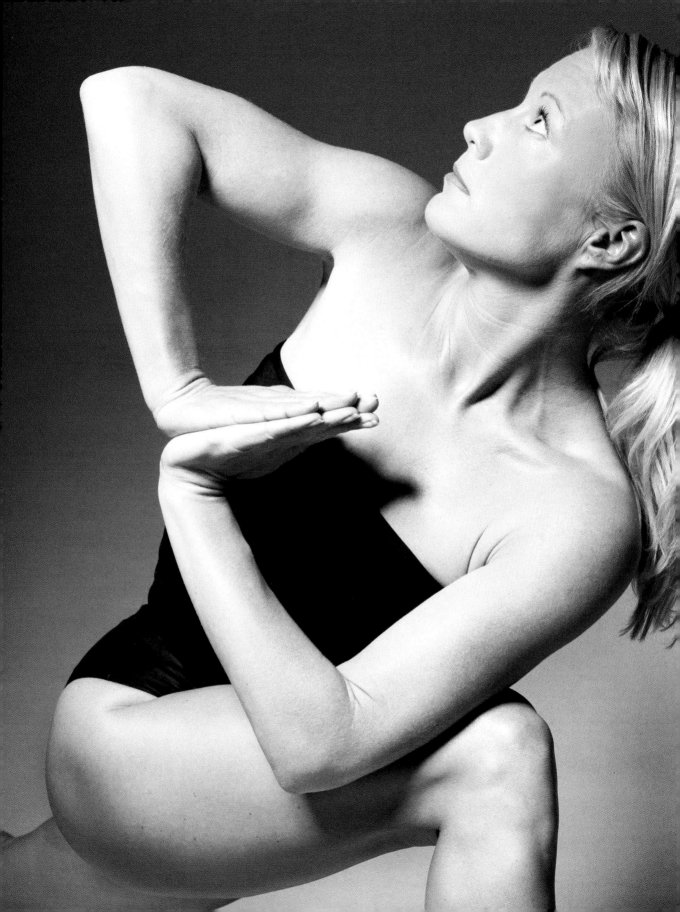

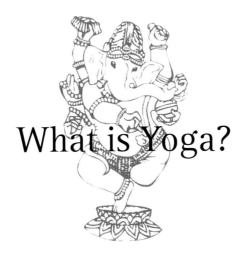

What is Yoga?

People generally used to believe yoga consisted solely of stretching exercises, mantra repetition, and breathing techniques. Today we know this isn't entirely true. The development of yoga over the last 5,000 years has aimed to help you cope with all of the physical, psychological, and spiritual trials in the surrounding world. You can achieve perfect health only if all the areas of your life are balanced. If you exercise with yoga, you can learn to create a balance between body, mind, and soul. Yoga gives you a calm, focused mind and a strong and flexible body. It also gives you a sense of unity, harmony, satisfaction, and peace of mind.

Yoga is one of the six basic schools in the Indian philosophy that together are called *darsana*: the way to see. Here yoga is described as an accurate and concrete metaphysical method to develop and create clarity in the way we perceive (and experience) ourselves. Yoga has many meanings, and they are all rooted in mobility and development. The word *yoga* means "to unite, join together." This union refers to the vertical band between body and soul that exists in all people. At the same time, it refers to the vertical band between the self and the true identity (*atman, purusha*). This band is also connected to Brahman, the universal energy, or soul. Yoga is often described as being based on the knowledge of life, and it can be seen as a platform where body, soul, and mind meet through mobility, breathing techniques, concentration, and body control. Yoga is based on universal laws, and it can be defined as the science of creating balance between body and soul, as well as between rest and activity. Yoga works on two levels:

1. It makes us stronger and fills up the energy depots so we can cope with more things in our lives. At the same time it helps us relax and rest.

2. It trains us in being present at any given moment, to remove the things that disturb our concentration and the things that restrict us and make us restless.

In his book *The Illustrated World's Religions*, Huston Smith describes yoga as a discipline that aims for integration and unification. The highest goal is to understand that the individual is part of a greater whole. When you practice yoga, it makes your identity stronger because you let go of stress, tension, and imbalances in the body that could lead to bad energy, poor knowledge of the self, poor health, and destructive behavior.

The mind is unpredictable and hard to master; it swings and dances through new activities. It is good to control the mind. A controlled mind creates happiness. — Buddha.

Is yoga a religion?

Yoga is often connected to Hinduism, Buddhism, or Jainism, but its roots can be found in the philosophical traditions of India. While it has some principles in common with Buddhist, Hindu, and Jain teachings, yoga is a system of thought—not a religion. It has no religious tradition and is better understood as a natural science that bases itself solely on personal experience. Yoga is a method to achieve awareness and to experience a higher consciousness through physical, mental, and spiritual development. Rather than interfering with a person's religious convictions, ideally it should strengthen them by adding broadened perspective to one's understanding. Religion encourages a collective mindset, while yoga adheres to the law of nature and life, as well as the thoughts and feelings of the individual. You don't have to believe in anything or anyone but yourself and your own development when you practice yoga. To the individual, yoga offers the possibility of a transformation that involves a quest for complete human fulfilment on all levels. This means that regardless of your personality, faith, or physical attributes, you can find the path that leads to maximum strength, vitality, and freedom.

Yoga types and paths

Yoga can be compared to a tree on which each single branch represents a certain movement or path. The most famous branches are *Tantra Yoga* (this is the oldest branch, "the main trunk"), *Bhakti Yoga* (devotion), *Jnana Yoga* (knowledge/wisdom), *Raja Yoga* (meditation/interspection), *Karma Yoga* (action), and *Hatha Yoga* (forceful physical yoga).

Tantra Yoga is the oldest path in yoga. Through tantric techniques, you can gradually learn to sense, understand, and see energy. This path works with the symbolic energy *shakti* (feminine energy) in order to evoke the *Kundalini*-power (the primordial power) that is located at the bottom of the spine. Tantra Yoga embraces all other paths in yoga. It sometimes uses the body to carry out different exercises and meditation. The purpose is to promote positive thoughts and become more conscious of sexual energy.

Bhakti Yoga. Bhakti means emotional devotion towards the divine. Bhakti Yoga is the path of love and devotion. This devotion is expressed in prayers, rituals, and ceremonial worshipping. You give praise to the divine in all of nature's creatures. This type of yoga focuses on worshipping the divinity you find in your own heart and mind.

Jnana Yoga. Jnana means wisdom and knowledge. This is the intellectual path in yoga. The goal here is to achieve a pure mind freed from shallowness and vanity. In Jnana Yoga, you create balance through trying to separate reality from illusion (*maya*) so that you can achieve clarity and strength.

Raja Yoga. Raja Yoga combines all branches of yoga, and it can include Karma, Jnana, and Bhakti. Raja means "royal," and Raja Yoga sees the body as a "vehicle" for spiritual energy. Raja Yoga primarily focuses on meditation and on consciously controlling the human mind. Raja Yoga arose due to the work of Patanjali and the text *Yoga Sutras*.

Karma Yoga. Karma means action. This branch of yoga works on achieving balance through unselfish actions (primarily through some sort of community service). Karma is suitable for people who have a calm and patient nature and who are interested in supporting and working with other people.

Hatha Yoga is often called "the path of the body" or "classical yoga." Hatha Yoga is a sequence of *asanas*, or poses, that train the body, soul, and mind. Hatha means "power" and "strength," but it also has a more esoteric meaning. In Sanskrit, *ha* means "solar" or masculine energy (yang), and *tha* means "lunar" or feminine energy (yin). Yoga refers to the unification of these two fundamental universal energies—the expanding energy of the sun and the contracting energy of the moon. These two forces can also be defined as two different directions; one of them goes out of the body, and the other goes into the body. These same energies keep the planets and the bodily organs in place. Ha is forceful and makes us robust, strong, focused, vigorous, firm, and productive. Tha makes us noble, extroverted, sensitive, loving, and capacious. According to classical physical yoga philosophy, you must discipline the body before you can achieve a disciplined mind. When we practice asanas, the masculine and feminine energies in all of us are combined and balanced. Yoga is knowledge of balance in everyday life, and it can help us master all the things we do. It can also teach us how to create harmony in our relationships with other people and understand our inner truth. Yoga exercises are divided into different types of asanas, Pranayama (breathing control), and Raj Asanas (meditative poses), as well as nauli, mudras, and bandhas (cleansing exercises). In the beginning the exercises might seem strange, but as you become more familiar with them, you will better understand how they work.

Hatha Yoga is an extension of Raja Yoga, but contains many tantric techniques as well. The text *Hatha Yoga Pradipika* by Svatmarama is the primary reference for this yogic path. Hatha Yoga is the basis of the development of many types of yoga during the last 100 to 150 years. In many yoga books written by well-known authors, it's explained that the reason for this is that yoga has always focused on strengthening and balancing the individual here and now. If we look at the history of yoga, it has always adjusted itself to the human being and its current environment. Even though many types of yoga focus on different solutions to the problem, all types of yoga have the same philosophical foundation. They stem from the same ancient scriptures about thought and physical structure. However, certain types of yoga are more oriented towards the physical aspects than others—for instance, *Vini Yoga*[3], *Ashtanga Vinyasa Yoga*[4], *Iyengar Yoga*[5], *Bikram Yoga*[6] and *Power Yoga* (also referred to as *Vinyasa Yoga*). These are all based on the general idea that all exercises ought to be done in one flowing movement. Other types of yoga, for instance *Kripali Yoga*[7] and *Kundalini Yoga*[8], are gentler.

Power Yoga is a dynamic style of Hatha Yoga. Many believe that it is the type of yoga that can most easily adjust to an individual's capabilities. It is primarily based on the Vini Yoga philosophy of *vinyasa-krama*, and it resembles the three steps in Kripali Yoga, in which you take one step at a time in order to achieve a flowing movement, strength, balance, mobility, and flexibility. Power Yoga has for a long time been an umbrella term for the dynamic types of yoga that derive from Vini Yoga. These types of yoga are vigorous and based on strength. At the end of the 1980s many yoga masters returned to the gentler type of Vini Yoga, and Power Yoga became an independent term. The popularity of Power Yoga has grown enormously over the last years, and the majority of its practitioners can be found in the United States, Western Europe, and Australia.

Highly concentrated breathing is the main focus. Here the aim is to integrate the yoga methods one step at a time[9]. Power Yoga is a vigorous type of yoga that demands you use your body and carry your own weight through a combination of movements, poses, and deep breaths. The power in yoga comes from working with *prana*, the life power energy. The more prana that flows along the spine, the more balanced, strong, and positive you feel. The flowing movements release energy, and, combined with the correct kind of breathing, your energy becomes vital and your mind grows more disciplined. Power Yoga builds up strength and focus, eliminates poisonous substances and waste products from the body, and reduces stress and tension in joints and muscles. As a result, imbalances in the body are reduced, and flexibility and mobility improve.

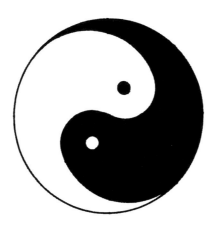

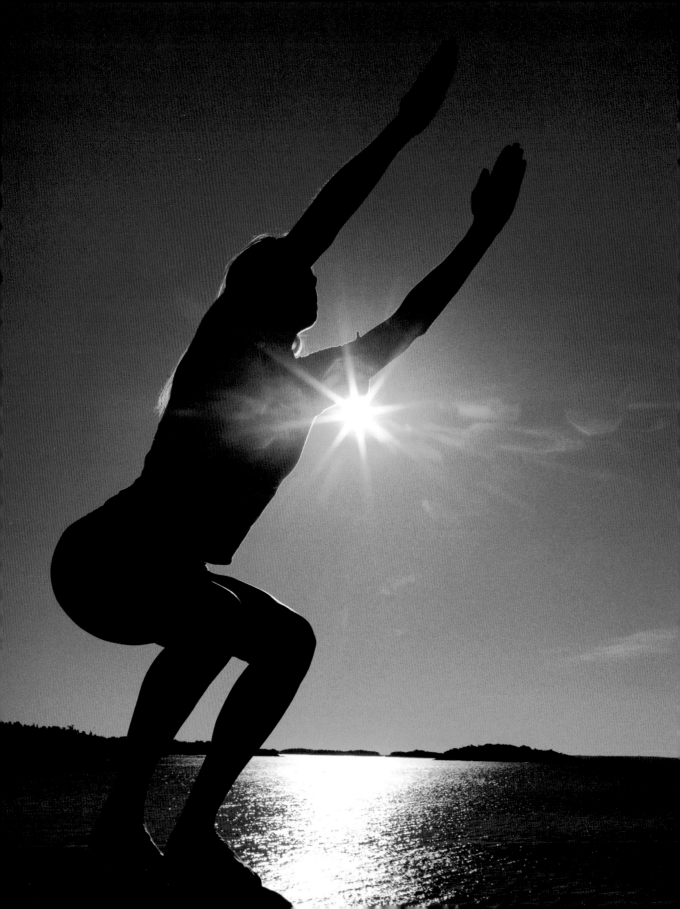

Progress can only be achieved through challenge. These exercises must take place at a speed that weighs the physical qualifications, the body history, and the thoughts and feelings of each individual. If you regularly do Power Yoga, you will often feel immediate results. Your intuition, mind, and body will get stronger, you will gain a deeper knowledge of bodily functions, become calmer, and in many cases lose weight. In Power Yoga, flexibility isn't the primary goal but rather an optimal feeling of strength, freedom, and vitality. This makes it suitable for all people, no matter their level of training. Your own physical abilities determine the intensity of the training, and because of this, Power Yoga is more open, free, accessible, and dynamic than the more "dogmatic" yoga types.

Sometimes Power Yoga is perceived negatively because of the misconception that it's an entirely new way to train without any basis in the ancient teachings of yoga. Power Yoga is a new branch in dynamic yoga, but its basic features and its idea of flowing movements and physical asanas (poses) can be traced back to the Vini Yoga tradition. Its philosophy derives from the philosophical Hindu document *Yoga Korunta* that some yoga scholars believe was found by the yoga master Shri Krishnamacharya in Northern India (more on page 33).

Power yoga as physical therapy

The movements in Power Yoga are as a whole well balanced, geared to develop strength and flexibility. The original idea of combining poses and movements with breathing makes the training life-affirming and physically challenging. The flowing structure and the breathing in Power Yoga make the body temperature go up. This heals the body; imbalances are reduced, it becomes easier to relax, and you get mentally and emotionally stronger.

As early as 600 BC, yoga was described as a spiritual attempt to control and calm the mind. It was believed that this was only possible through serious training and being present in the moment. Patanjali claims in *Yoga Sutras* that yoga is a suspension of, or a break in, the mind's thought waves, known as *vrittis*. You can learn how to control these thought waves when you do physical asanas and dynamic breathing. Yoga isn't about change; it is about constant awareness, focus, and presence in the moment. When you concentrate on movement and breathing, it is hard to think of anything else without losing concentration. As long as you keep the body in a flowing movement and use breathing as an "engine," your mind becomes stronger, and the mind melts into the physical body and is united with it.

Five thousand years ago a theory arose that the body can't be stretched when it is cold. It has to be warmed up before and during the exercises. This is why movements and poses that strengthen and warm up the muscles are combined. This is possible because breathing is directly linked to the nervous system that controls all our muscles. Without using strength in training, the heat won't spread to the muscles, and the exercises will not be efficient, safe, or possible to carry out. Sports and athletic activity alone can't keep us fit. Far too often such training makes the muscular system tense, and imbalances are created due to uneven use of the muscular groups or one-sided training (using one side of the body more than the other). Most sports injuries occur because of structural or muscular imbalances, and they don't heal themselves. One would assume cross training is a viable solution, and while it's better than one-sided training, it doesn't prevent injuries, heal them, or create bodily balance. If an imbalance occurs as a result of training in a certain sport, it doesn't get better from continuing to practice the same sport. Rest can to a certain extent heal injuries, but it doesn't change what caused the problem. The same imbalance will return, and the injury can come back. To heal physical imbalances and injuries, the muscular tissue must be worked on in different ways; through stretching as well as through contraction. This requires heat.

Power Yoga is a type of yoga that builds up strength and endurance. The movements generate a lot of heat, and you often sweat during the exercises, especially when you get used to—and master—correct breathing. It is exactly the heat that is generated in training that makes yoga efficient physical therapy. See yourself as a glassblower in his workshop. The glassblower takes his iron pipe, dips it in sand, puts it in the oven and then blows in to the iron pipe, and the red-hot lump expands into a bubble. The glassblower is now able to shape the bubble as he pleases, but he has to have constant access to heat or else the bubble will stiffen. He can't work on the bubble if it is cooled down because then it turns into glass that easily breaks. A chemical process takes place. The heat helps the circulation. Our bodies in yoga training work in the same way. The combination of breathing and specific poses helps to eliminate waste products, and the body system is revitalized. Nutrition is consumed, poisons eliminated, the organs are cleansed and massaged, and the muscular tissue is strengthened and rebuilt. Power Yoga builds up strength, energy, and heat through focusing, concentration, breathing, and doing exercises that help you learn how to control the functions of the autonomic nervous system. You learn how to control the pulse, the muscles, and the brain waves. Power Yoga gives you increased stamina because the active physical training increases the absorption of oxygen into the lungs. The breathing technique lowers the heart rhythm even though the exercises might feel exhausting. Yoga's impact on heart and lungs is the same as aerobic exercise: your resting pulse is lowered, and oxygen absorption is increased. Power Yoga concentrates on personal strength, as well as helping you learn how to listen to, and work with, yourself.

In Power Yoga, resting is just as important as the physical part of your training. The two work together to create optimal balance. If the mind is strained, stress, anxiety, uneasiness, tension, injuries, discomfort, and stiffness will be the result. If you do Power Yoga on a regular basis, it becomes easier to handle stress and gain new perspectives on many of life's difficult situations. Power Yoga gives you self-control, and it gives you power and strength to emancipate yourself from stress, uneasiness, anxiety, uncertainty, and mood swings. This is only possible if you let go of the idea of perfection, performance, and results. It takes time, training, and focus, but you will get better much sooner than you think!

The *Bhagavad-Gita* from around 300 to 400 BC contains many thoughts and ideas about self-realization. Here it is written that the soul is connected to our five senses, but first and foremost to our vision and our hearing. What we see and hear creates feelings, such as acknowledgement or disapproval, temptation or escape, that influence how we react. Too many impressions mean we can't sort out our feelings in a calm and thoughtful way. The soul is left out. That leads to a sense of inner emptiness and weakness, which limits our ability to appreciate the moment and live life to the fullest.

In yoga, focusing, *drishti*, trains the eyes, fixing them on a certain point to keep your thoughts from running loose. The purpose is to keep the energy inside you. Additionally, you train your hearing to listen exclusively to your own breathing (and quite often to pleasant music) when you do yoga exercises. It is exactly the flowing movements and the dynamic breathing in Power Yoga that make it easier for you to concentrate on the moment you're in. The mind gets stronger, and the soul can express itself.

Yoga asanas as injury prevention

Stiffness almost always occurs along the back of the body, and tense, stiff muscles can lead to tiredness, weakness, aggression, headaches, injuries, and negative thoughts. Physical yoga softens and reduces muscular tension and makes the muscles longer and stronger. When tension in muscles and joints is relaxed, *emotional release* takes place. It's not unusual for people to start crying, sweating, or freezing when they relax in *Corpse Pose* at the end of their physical exercises. Something positive happens when the body releases its reserves of tension and negative stress so that it can be strengthened in the moment and absorb the power that is inside every one of us. Also, the body can remind us if there is an imbalance in our soul. If you have blocked out a negative experience, it will only be hidden beneath other unpleasant experiences. The body has a cellular memory, and everything you have done or experienced is stored inside its DNA. The body never forgets anything. When you physically open your body, negative stress and tension (in muscles, cells, and muscular tissue) are reduced.

When we speak of injuries, we usually refer to two kinds: acute injuries (for example, a bone fracture) and chronic injuries, which stem from overstraining yourself, one-sided movement patterns, or, in many cases, psychosomatic causes. A lot of chronic injuries can be healed and prevented with yoga. The most common injuries, like knee problems that are caused by weakness in the quadriceps (thigh muscles) or one-sided rigorous training, can be helped through static training and strength training, combined with dynamic stretching exercises and mobility training. All these elements can be achieved when you do Power Yoga. Runner's knees or hip injuries, sciatica, inflammation of the periosteum; injuries, soreness, or stiffness on the back of the thighs; inflammation of the Achilles' tendon; heel spur; calf or ankle strains; stress fractures; minor hip problems; shoulder injuries; neck and back problems; intestine problems and certain metabolism problems—all these disorders can be diminished or disappear completely if you regularly practice Power Yoga. If you suffer from any of these imbalances or injuries while you are doing Power Yoga (or other types of yoga), it is important to start slowly and be aware of how far you can go into the exercises. Build up the training slowly.

Yoga can be characterized as active rest, and you can do yoga every day without damaging your body. I myself have benefited from using yoga in treating injuries that were caused by other types of sports and training. I quickly got rid of physical injuries including inflammation of the Achilles' tendon, problems after knee injuries (straining of a ligament), runner's knees, intestine imbalances, and neck problems.

The physical influence of yoga

Yoga is different from other types of exercise and training first and foremost because it isn't competitive. Yoga is about constantly being aware of the development of your body. It is about listening to your body instead of forcing it to do things it is not ready for, which can only lead to frustration and, in the worst cases, injuries. In yoga exercises, the muscles are stretched to their full length, and from that they gain stamina. The fat around the cells disappears and, in combination with the right breathing techniques, the exercises improve circulation and promote the elimination of poisonous substances. This process is especially useful if you have cellulite. Yoga exercises have a positive effect on the thyroid gland that regulates metabolism, and regularly doing yoga can help you reach and stay at your ideal weight. Yoga also builds up your immune defences as it trains and strengthens the inner organs so that your body can work like a car in tiptop shape. When you do deep stretching, strength exercises, and use the right breathing techniques, yoga counteracts the physical tension and softens the muscular stiffness that often causes illnesses, difficulties, and bad moods. When you train the physical body using concentration, focus, and breathing, you create a strong and long lasting sense of harmony in the body, mind, and soul.

Food and life style

Many people think that when you practice yoga, you also have to change all your old habits. You don't have to say no to alcohol, meat, or cigarettes just because you practice yoga! Yoga is not about being ascetic but about moderation. Yoga is about letting the body return to its natural balance, and after training a while you will have achieved the necessary energy to do so. When mind and body are in harmony, and when you are centered in yourself, you'll *want* to maintain a healthy life style. Some people choose to exercise yoga to the fullest, while others just use yoga as part of everyday life. A lot of people are content staying where it feels emotionally comfortable for them, while others choose a deeper and more arduous spiritual path to find answers, knowledge, and deeper understanding. We all have our own goals, feelings, thoughts, and bodies, so why shouldn't we practice yoga in different ways? Yoga allows you to develop at a pace that's best suited for you.

[3] *Vini Yoga was developed by Shri Krishnamacharya and was further developed by his son T.K.V. Desikachar. A recognized teacher of B.K.S. Iyengar, Shri K. Pattabhi Jois, and Indra Devi, Shri Krishnamacharya introduced a renaissance of Hatha Yoga that led to a development in yoga up through the 20th century. Vini Yoga works with what we call "sequence process" or* vinyasa-krama. *Here the emphasis is not placed on physically perfect poses but rather on the conditions and needs of the one who practices yoga. The coordination of movement and breathing is an important aspect of Vini Yoga.*

[4] *Ashtanga Vinyasa Yoga was developed by K. Pattabhi Jois, who was a student of Shri Krishnamacharya. This type of yoga is very athletic and strenuous, and runs in three sequences. You have to master the first sequence perfectly before you move on to the next if you want to achieve the maximum effect. It is acrobatic, and from the start it demands a lot when it comes to muscle strength and physical capability. Terminology from Sanskrit is used during training, and the pace is fairly high. Both Iyengar and Ashtanga Yoga are contemporary types of yoga that have developed from Hatha Yoga during the 20th century.*

[5] *Iyengar Yoga was developed by B.K.S. Iyengar who was the brother-in-law of Shri Krishnamacharya. This style was developed around the same time as Ashtanga Yoga, and is characterized by precision training using tools like pillows, wooden blocks, sand bags, and belts. It is sometimes called 'furniture yoga.' The exercise in itself contains different sequences of standing, seated and bending poses, and the emphasis is placed on strength, precision, flexibility, and perfect posture. Iyengar Yoga demands that you are in good basic condition, that you are relatively flexible, and have a lot of energy and strength.*

[6] *This is a fairly new yoga style developed by Bikram Choudhury. It contains 26 asanas, exercised in standard sequences in a room set at 104 degrees (Fahrenheit). This system requires a strong physique. Bikram Yoga has become very popular among the rich and famous in Hollywood.*

[7] *This three-step yoga type was developed by Yogi Amrit Desai, a student of Kripalvananda. The first step is about body posture and the coordination of breathing and movement. You do the different poses over a relatively short time span. In the second step, meditation is integrated in the training, and the poses are held a little longer. In the third and last step, the training of asanas has become a spontaneous meditation in motion.*

[8] *This is another basic type of yoga in which body and soul are equally important. The word* kundalini *can be translated into the primordial power that shall be woken and stimulated by simple but dynamic yoga movements combined with breathing—and concentration exercises. The emphasis is placed on endurance. It is an independent yoga type developed by the Sikh teacher Yogi Bhajan.*

[9] *It is better for your health to make the asanas fit the practitioner than the other way around.*

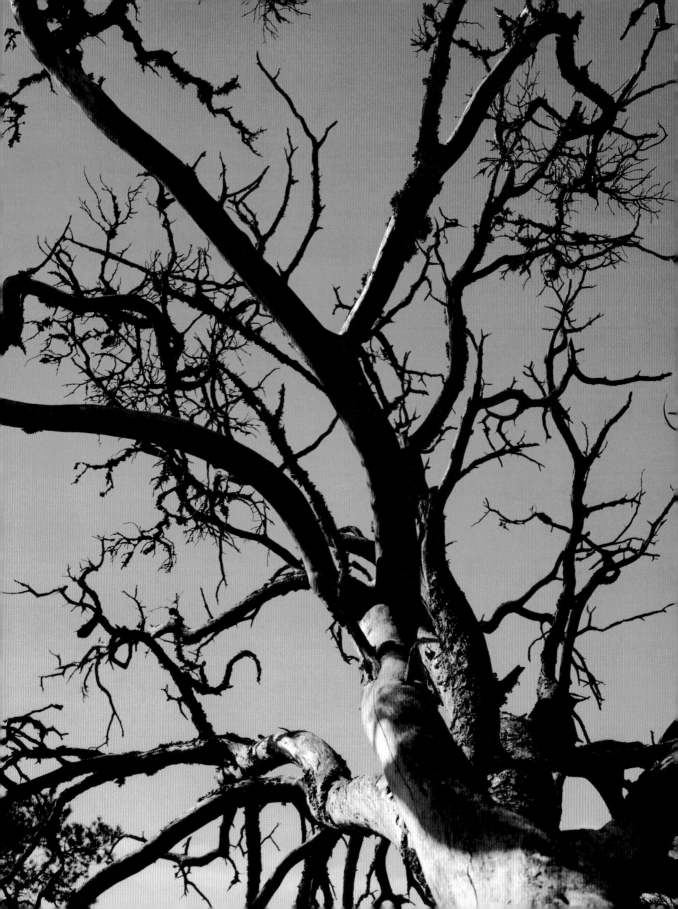

Back to the Roots

Through aspiring, hard work, discipline and controlling the self, the wise man can create for himself an island that no river, no sea, is able to sink or flood. — Buddha

Yoga's history can be traced back thousands of years. The oldest evidence comes from archaeological finds from the earliest civilization in the Indus Valley. This advanced culture developed on the banks of the Indus River in Northern India bordering Pakistan, and it covered an area of hundreds of miles from the north to the south. Throughout the many archaeological finds in this area, not a single weapon was found. It's possible these people were more peaceful than other civilizations, or they might have been practitioners of one of yoga's moral concepts, *ahimsa*[10]. Excavations in Mohenjo-Dara and Harappa, the biggest cities of this civilization, hundreds of small terracotta figurines and inscriptions believed to be more than 4,000 years old were found.

In *Health, Healing & the Living Tradition of Krishnamacharya*, T.K.V. Desikachar writes that one of the many yoga teachers he trained once had the opportunity to study and investigate these figurines and inscriptions. He found images of the Hindu god Shiva meditating in a sophisticated lotus pose called the *mulabandhasana*. Though this is an interesting discovery, we don't know whether yoga was an active part of these peoples' lives. Most scientists claim that yoga didn't exist as a fully developed and complex tradition before 500 BC.

Yoga's history

Deeper insight into yoga's historical and philosophical origins can be found in the old Indian scriptures the *Vedas*, the *Upanishads*, the *Bhagavad-Gita*, *Yoga Sutras*, and *Yoga Korunta*. The modern yoga teacher Georg Feuerstein has arranged the historical map of yoga into five paths:

Vedic Yoga. In the *Vedas*, you can find the oldest written traces of Indian culture and yoga. The Vedas are a three thousand year old collection of hymns and rituals that suggest a strong ritual life in the early Indian civilization. Vedic Yoga, also called *Archaic Yoga*, focuses on the idea of making sacrifices: you, as an individual, should learn how to unite the visible physical and material worlds with the invisible spiritual world. To practice these rituals and sing these hymns in the proper way, you have to focus and concentrate thoughts and emotions in your mind for a certain time span. The Vedic philosophy, passed on by so-called *rishis*, was available not only to priests, monks, astrologists, astronomers, or other members of the religious elite, but to the layperson as well. The hymns of Vedic prophets bear witness to a strong intuition, wisdom, and insight that today can inspire us to further understand human life, development, and evolution.

Preclassical Yoga. The central yoga literature from 600 to 800 BC is the *Upanishads*. They are the esoteric continuation of the Vedic rituals. The Upanishads are a collection of texts that deal with metaphysical speculations. Like the Vedas, they are regarded as mysterious revelations. In contrast to the more open and popular scriptures from the Vedic period, the Upanishads were secret scriptures. Some of these two hundred Gnostic texts are directly related to yoga and express a complete solidarity with all living things. At this point, yoga started forming and its secret philosophy spread from teacher to student, and not from Rishis to the people as was the case in the Vedic period. The concept of an individual system of thoughts came into being.

The most famous and popular text in both yoga and Hindu literature is the *Bhagavad-Gita*, which was written around 300 to 400 BC. *Bhagavad-Gita* is the fictional tale of a conversation between the Hindu god Krishna and Prince Arjuna. Ironically, the action takes place on a battlefield; however, this is often seen as a metaphor for the chaotic world that constantly calls for our attention. Arjuna finds himself in a difficult situation for which he only can blame himself. He has to go to war and fight against some of his friends who are on the enemy's side, so he invokes Krishna for advice and guidance. Symbolically, this frustration is all about how he can cut his ties to the material world and free himself and his spirit. Krishna says that it's Arjuna's job to handle this situation, but that he can be victorious if he follows a detailed yoga path. This path goes through devotion (*Bhakti Yoga*), acuteness (*Jnana Yoga*), and unselfish action (*Karma Yoga*), which would then allow Arjuna to achieve spiritual liberation (*moksha*). *Bhagavad-Gita* is a complex book that rewards those who read, study, and meditate on its meaning.

Classical yoga. This period covers the Eight-Fold Path Yoga that is described in *Yoga Sutras* by Patanjali. This text, written in Sanskrit, contains approximately 196 aphorisms (short thoughts of wisdom) that have been commented on a good many times since they were published sometime around the 5th century. Yoga Sutras depicts yoga in a systematic way and is regarded by many yogis (people who practice yoga) to be the fundamental source of yogi understanding. Literally the word *sutra*[11] means 'thread,' but in this context it means the thread of *recollection*. This 'thread' symbolically reminds the reader to be attentive to the knowledge of the wise Patanjali and the wisdom in the texts. Today, we know very little about Patanjali except that he believed that every individual was made of matter (*prakriti*) and soul (*purusha*). This philosophical dualism is important, since most of the Indian philosophical systems are concerned either with matter *or* soul—non-dualism. In the first book of the *Yoga Sutra*, yoga is defined as "a stop in the thought-waves of the mind" (*citta vritti nirodha*). In *The Heart of Yoga*, T.K.V. Desikachar describes yoga as "the ability to direct the mind exclusively toward an object and sustain that direction without any distractions." These thought-waves in the mind, called *vrittis*, are often referred to as "monkey mind." This analogy describes how the untrained mind jumps around from branch to branch without ever stopping. Practicing yoga is seen as an attempt to focus the mind on one point—without distraction or interruption—in order to calm and stabilize the wild monkey.

The eight paths described in *Yoga Sutra* are: *yama*—moderation, humility; *niyama*—observation; *asana*—posture, mobility; *pranayama*—breathing, energy control; *pratyahara*—

abduction of the mind; *dharana*—concentration; *dhyana*—meditation; *samadhi*—happiness or complete insight.

The first path, *yama*, implies a sort of preparatory moral to inspire the yogi. *Yama* is based on five fundamentals that together are seen as the foundation of the entire yoga discipline and the basis of mental growth. They are the ethical ground that yoga philosophy builds itself upon, but they are very complex and impossible to follow completely.

1. *Ahimsa*, or non-violence. It is impossible to live without any sort of violence. None of us can live a perfect life without at some point using violence towards others or ourselves. In this moral demand, Patanjali says that if it is possible, you should avoid using violence or behaving in an aggressive manor. Such behavior will only lead to imbalances. The purpose of ahimsa is to become humble towards all living creatures. The only way you can possibly carry out ahimsa in everyday life is to be aware of how violence and negative feelings interfere in your own life. It is a self-contradiction if you present yourself as a non-violent person, then throw red paint on people who wear fur, or buy a hamburger or a pair of leather shoes. Ahimsa is all about being kind, compassionate, understanding, patient, and loving. It is, however, important to emphasize that this should count in all actions, towards yourself as well as towards others. It also doesn't mean that after one day of performing kind actions you can tell yourself: "I'm the best human being in the world!" to drown out possible feelings of low self-esteem. Many people in modern society have low self-esteem, and one of the ways we can become stronger is to reflect upon the idea of non-violence by thinking: what kind of thoughts do I have about myself? What am I saying to myself? Am I really that bad? Would I ever say to other people what I say to myself? Another way we can relate to non-violence is to remind ourselves that all living creatures love life. Look at birds, insects, fish, and mammals. They guard their lives and always fly away from the things that hunt them. A human life is not more sacred than others. We are all part of the ecosystem, and each single organism is necessary in the circle of life. This idea might provoke some, but the goal is to form your own understanding of things.

2. *Satya*, or *truth*. A human being should seek to live life in truth. To be true to oneself. To speak the truth out of love, and not because you're forced to.

3. *Asteya*, or *not to steal*. Patanjali has said that if you want to be liberated and feel happy, you should not take something that doesn't belong to you if that thing isn't offered

to you. He doesn't only speak of material things. Time, emotions, energy, thoughts, and ideas can be stolen, too. Buddha said that at the end of our spiritual journey we "throw everything back." By this he meant that we live in a material world, but when we gain insight and become wiser, the material world isn't as important anymore. He believes that if we mirror ourselves in our possessions and all the material things we see around us, we can't see our true selves.

4. *Aparigraha*, or *not to collect*. The basic thought in yoga is to live in the present. That's very difficult when we take into consideration all the things that exist around us and all the things we have to do. The biggest problem of our time seems to be different kinds of burdens. There is too much information to process: Web sites, technology, work projects, financial opportunities. There is too much that has to be done, seen, and experienced. Patanjali encourages us to simplify our mantra. We could stop buying unnecessary things, and ask ourselves if we really need a new carpet, a vase, or new clothes. He doesn't suggest an ascetic and boring life, but rather suggests you should start thinking about whether or not you really need all the material stuff you surround yourself with. Patanjali believes that if we build our lives solely on material possessions, we aren't free.

5. *Brahmacharya*, or *moderation*. This is about the core of energy within you. Some scholars refer to it as your relationship to the divine; others say that it refers to your relationship to nature. When you reflect upon Bracmacharya, you should pay attention to what you spend your energy on and how you spend it. According to the Yoga Sutras, you should try to avoid superficial thoughts and not use energy on people, systems, or business that only *take* your energy without giving anything back. You should try to balance both outgoing and inward coming energy. To achieve this, you have to ask yourself: who am I? How am I doing? What makes me feel good or bad? Why do I feel bad when I do certain things or meet certain people? Think about it, and think about the answers you come up with. For some people this will lead to a time of dissociation so they can put everything into perspective.

According to Patanjali, there are four paths that lead to self-realization, liberation, and a stronger self: love, recognition, work, and psychophysical training. After practicing the yoga methods, you feel filled with love, harmony, and peace, and it takes a lot after that to feel the urge to steal or be violent. The meaning of "unity" in yoga is all about the melting together of body, mind, and soul. In order to truly understand how this alliance is made possible, you have to pay attention to the physical structure of yoga, its breathing and the way it works with *prana*, life energy. Body and soul are already united, and they share life in us but on an unconscious level. Yoga makes it possible to see and respect each single part of the body as part of a unity. Yoga also makes it possible to experience the strength of each single part, so that you can become a stronger, more open and balanced individual. The system of yoga makes this alliance visible.

Postclassical Yoga. A couple of hundred years after Patanjali, yoga took an interesting turn. In the time that followed *Yoga Sutras*, many new schools of yoga came into being. During this period, the goal was to achieve complete solidarity with all living things. Now the focus was put on the possibilities of the human body. Prior generations of yogis—or yoga masters—were more interested in self-absorption and meditation, and their goal was to leave the body and the world in order to unite with the formless reality— the soul. But the period that followed found inspiration in alchemy, chemistry's philosophical predecessor. A new generation of yogis developed a system in which different exercises that included breathing and meditation would lead to rejuvenation of the body and thereby prolong life. The body was now seen as a temple for the immortal soul and not just a container you could leave when the opportunity arose. By using advanced yoga techniques, they investigated the possibility of achieving optimal energy and strength. These developments led to the creation of Hatha Yoga and the different paths and schools in Tantra Yoga.

Modern Yoga. Modern yoga has its roots in an 1893 conference at *The Parliament of Religions* in Chicago, Illinois. During this meeting the young Swami Vivekananda from India left a deep impression when he talked about yoga philosophy and history. He became one of the most popular members of the parliament, and he lectured on yoga all over America. After Swami[12] Vivekananda, many yoga masters crossed the ocean and lectured across the country. Yoga schools were founded, and more and more people saw the potential in yoga. Many went to Europe too, but they weren't equally welcomed there.

Hatha Yoga had its debut in America when the Russian born yogi Indra Devi, often called "the grand lady of yoga," opened a yoga studio in Hollywood in 1947. She taught movie stars like Gloria Swanson, Jennifer Jones, and Robert Ryan, and she educated hundreds of yoga trainers. In the 1950s, one of the most prominent yoga teachers, Selvarajan Yesudian, wrote the book *Sport and Yoga*, which introduced the yoga world to sports. The book has been translated into many languages and sold more than half a million copies.

In 1961, Richard Hittleman introduced Hatha Yoga on TV, and his book *The Twenty-Eight Day Yoga Plan* sold millions of copies. In the 1960s and the 1970s, yoga became a lifestyle, one largely adopted by the hippie movement. His Holiness the Dalai Lama is a great yogi from Tibet who represents Buddhism and Tibetan Yoga. As an advocate for peace, he received the Nobel Peace Prize in 1989, and throughout the 1980s and 1990s, he inspired many westerners to learn more about Tibetan Buddhism and yoga. The popularity of yoga has grown dramatically in recent years, and today more than 30 million people all over the world practice yoga. Now, yoga is part of a training regimen in many sports and by many sports teams (the Chicago Bulls are a famous example). It is now the fastest growing movement in health and fitness.

Yoga Korunta

The great yoga master and highly esteemed Sanskrit professor Krishnamacharya spent most of his life traveling throughout India. He demonstrated and lectured on yoga and on Hindu philosophy. While doing research in The National Archives of India, he found the ancient document *Yoga Korunta*. The manuscript was bound, and the paper was made from different kinds of leaves. He started studying the text and found a long and detailed chapter about Hatha Yoga written in Sanskrit[13] by a prophet called *Vamana Rishi*.

Krishnamacharya was understandably delighted upon finding this document, and after studying it, he discovered it was more than fifteen hundred years old. Linguistically, though, it was related to the oral tradition of classical Sanskrit, which is believed to be close to five thousand years old. These scriptures had been verbally passed on earlier, from teacher to student, throughout many generations. *Yoga Korunta* contains hundreds of verses structured in so-called metric sutras or phrases that resemble the ones found in *Yoga Sutra*. The first part of the scripture is about movements, or poses, and it explains the breathing technique in detail and what it takes to be able to do the movement or the pose to the fullest. The other part contains information about certain breathing techniques and reveals good advice on how you can develop on your own and become sufficiently strong, balanced, and concentrated in order to raise the level of performance. This advice had, up to this point, been kept secret. *Yoga Korunta* also deals with the notion that the highest possible amount of energy, freedom, and sense of vitality can be achieved exclusively through flowing movements and poses using dynamic breathing as an "engine." Each individual must perform in accordance with his own abilities and take one step at a time. *Yoga Korunta* is today seen as a "bible" to people who practice Vini Yoga (a type of yoga that was developed by Krishnamacharya) and its subgroups: Ashtanga Vinyasa Yoga, Iyengar Yoga, and Power Yoga.

[10] *Not to use violence or do harm (to yourself as well as to other people, nature, animals or other living creatures).*
[11] *Sutra is Sanskrit and related to the Latin* suture = stitch, seam.
[12] Swami *means master.*
[13] *According to both Western and Eastern research, Sanskrit is not only the world's oldest language but also the oldest language that is still spoken today. Even though Sanskrit is usually linked with India and its history, there is a connection between Sanskrit and modern European languages. Sanskrit was a forerunner of both Greek and Latin, and many words in both languages have their roots in Sanskrit. It is still uncertain, though, whether European languages really descended from Sanskrit or whether they together descend from an even older common family of languages. The type of Sanskrit that is spoken today is called classical Sanskrit and has been used for approximately 2,500 years.*

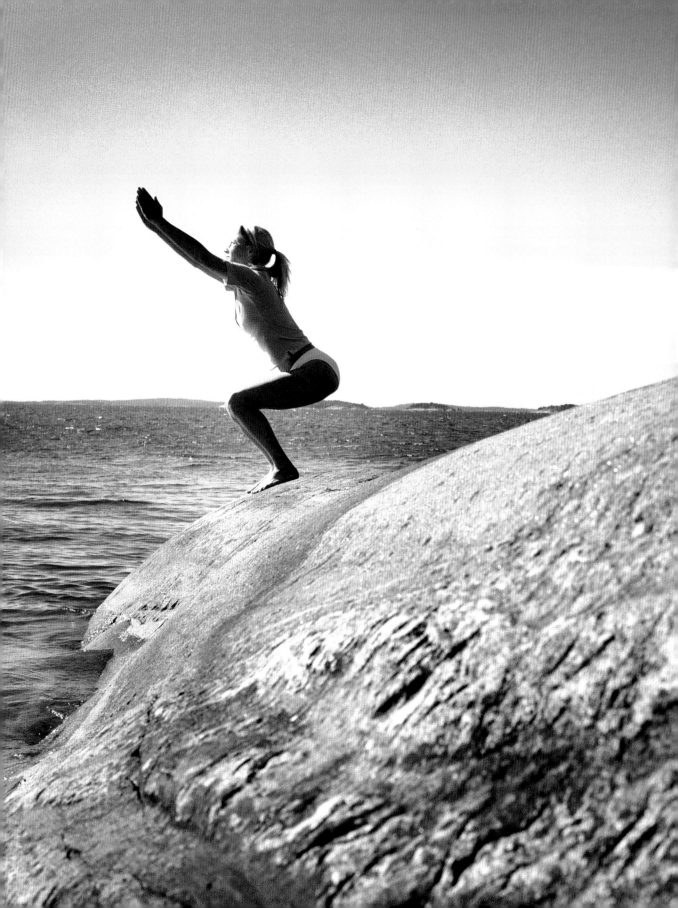

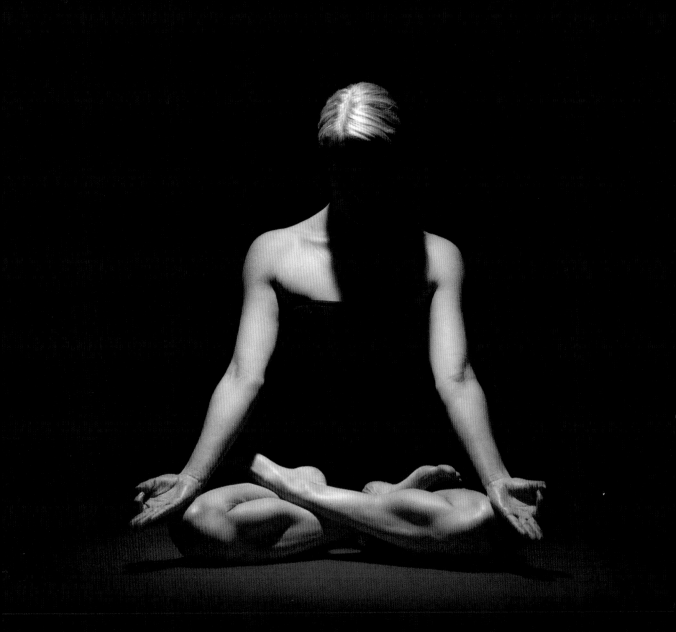

The Energy System

The physical body is filled with and surrounded by an electromagnetic field, a sort of bodily power station that stores and generates energy. You can't gain more energy, but the energy can be converted and transformed in a positive or a negative direction. This power station can be seen as an energy system that embraces the seven energy centers of the body called *chakras*[14] (there is an additional eighth chakra I'll return to later on in this chapter). Based in a belief system whose roots can be traced as far back as 4,000 years, the chakras are located along the spine, from the Root Chakra at the floor of the pelvis (*perineum*), to the top of the head where the Crown Chakra is located. The word "chakra" means "nerve center" ("circle of light" in Hindi), and they are often depicted like wheels. These nerve centers work like generators that regulate, store, and supply the body with *prana*—life power or life energy (subtle energy). On the spine, they cross the zones in which different *nadis* (channels along the spine that transport prana) meet, and here they create fields of energy, circles of light that vibrate and rotate on different frequencies depending on how much energy floats inside the circles.

The chakra system works much like a water mill. The water wheel spins faster the stronger the water stream is, and vice versa. The wheel spins when the energy (the water) is supplied, and the movement of the wheel starts to grind the corn. The chakra system works in the same way, but it uses prana instead of water and a center of energy instead of a wheel. The chakras can't be seen with the naked eye, but their locations along the spine correspond to a nerve center in the central nervous system. The chakras can be compared to databases that contain information that can't be seen in the physical world. These databases store the information (thoughts, feelings, instincts, memories, impressions, etc.) that are necessary for our reproduction and survival.

The first chakra, *Muladhara Chakra*, is at the end of the spine right above the anus, and it coincides with the wickerwork of nerves in the sacrum (*plexus sacralis*)[15], as well as with the adrenal glands that activate the body. This chakra is seen as the anchor of the bodily energy system. *Mula* means root or source in Sanskrit, and *adhara* means support or vital part. According to yoga teachings, this chakra is dominated by the earth element, and it is the body center that symbolizes our survival instinct and sense of security. The Root Chakra is the source of the need to own, conquer, compete, and collect things. Horror, insecurity, and the need for close contact stem from this chakra. When the Root

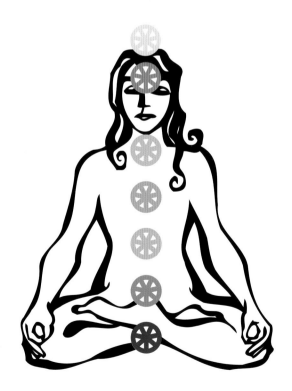

Chakra, which is connected to the color red, is balanced and filled with prana, a sense of peace, security, and grounding is released.

The second chakra, *Svadhisthana Chakra*, meaning "your origin," is right above the sexual glands. This chakra, which is connected to the color orange, coincides with the lumbar region or the hypo-gastric area (the lower part of the stomach or abdominal cavity). It coincides with the wickerwork of nerves in the sexual glands and the prostate (*plexus prostaticus*). It is also connected to the sexual glands that regulate our sexual instincts and activities. *Sva* means "your own" and *adhisthana* means "origin" or "source" in Sanskrit. The Svadhisthana Chakra is dominated by the water element, and it symbolizes creative energy. Here the source of physical, sexual, and creative energy is found, and the chakra is home to the origin of life, as well as the will and ability to reproduce. When prana flows in this chakra, unlimited love and creativity are at your disposal. If the opposite is the case, you might experience jealousy, anger, sexual insecurity, and dependency.

Manipura Chakra is the third chakra. Associated with the color yellow or gold, it's in the area around the navel and overlaps the *solar plexus*, the pancreas (*plexus solaris*), which regulates your blood sugar, and the wickerwork of nerves behind the pancreas. *Mani* means "jewel" and *puram* "city," or, more literally, the realm where your inner force (your "shining jewel") is located. From here, energy shoots upwards and sends light and heat (the fire element dominates this chakra) into the body. It is the body's center of strength, expression, and expansion. When a lot of prana circulates in this center, you can get to know your true self, but if there is little prana to be found here, selfish actions take place. The diaphragm, the muscle in the pit of the stomach, is placed in this area, and it is here that the body generates the most heat to organs, muscles, and other parts of the body. In Japanese martial arts, this center is called *hara*: "the place of strength."

The chakra controlled by the element of air is *Anahata Chakra*, which means "constant, new power." This chakra can be found in the area around the heart. The fourth chakra is connected to the heart and lung center and overlaps the wickerwork of nerves in the heart (*plexus cardiacus*) as well as the thymus gland[16]. Anahata Chakra is the center of compassion, unconditional love, humility, and forgiveness. When this area is filled with life force, you feel love for all living creatures no matter their origin, shape, color, or race. Advanced yogis often focus on this area when they meditate. They do this to gain insight into the life that goes on in their own bodies as well as outside it, and to be filled with new strength, energy, and love. This chakra is represented by the color green.

The fifth chakra is called *Vishuddha Chakra* (meaning "purest among everything pure"). It is characterized by the element of ether[17]. This neck chakra, symbolized by the color turquoise or blue, overlaps the wickerwork of nerves in the neck *(plexus cervicalis)* and is located on the same line that connects the throat/pharynx area. This neck chakra affects the thyroid gland, which regulates metabolism. It is seen as the door to wealth and freedom or liberation and independence. When there's balance in this chakra, we are emancipated from all impurity—anger, bitterness, and displeasure—and can enjoy unlimited independence. Speech becomes clearer, and according to yoga teachings, you can become a skilled lecturer and teacher.

The Forehead Chakra, or *Ajna Chakra*, represented by the color indigo (or in some yoga literature magenta), means "the third eye, inner consciousness" in Sanskrit. It can be found between the eyebrows and is signified by soul and thought. The Forehead Chakra covers the wickerwork of nerves in a vein in the skull *(plexus cavernosus)* as well as the pituitary gland—the gland that controls other hormonal glands. This center is said to control both incoming and outgoing thoughts. According to yoga philosophy, the third eye is the vertical eye of certainty that gives you the ability to unite the horizontal physical reality and the vertical spiritual level. That means that you can achieve a general idea of your own personality and its nature.

Finally, we have the highest placed chakra—the Crown Chakra or *Sahasrara Chakra*, *which* means "thousands of petals." This chakra, signified by the element of light, is connected to the cerebral center and the pineal gland, which is said to control sleep and waking. The Crown Chakra is represented by the color violet (or no color/white in some yoga literature) and a lotus flower with thousands of petals. When there's a high dose of prana in the Crown Chakra, it is symbolized in rays of light shining from the middle of the chakra. When meditating on this area, you might feel as if you are melting together with the universal energy. If you find yourself at this stage, you can achieve the highest insight, and there will be no division between "the self" and "everything else"—you become part of the present.

In yoga philosophy, prana wanders higher and higher up through the chakra system during our physical, psychological, and spiritual growth. The chakras are often split up into the three above and the three below the heart chakra. The heart chakra is itself the connecting link. This doesn't mean that the upper chakras are superior to the lower ones. It only means that the lower chakras vibrate on a lower frequency than the upper ones. When we practice yoga, this system is put into motion through concentration, focus, breathing, and exercises. Prana flows into the Root Chakra, and it then slowly starts spinning faster. This rotation makes prana elevate to the next chakra. The lower chakras have to rotate on the same frequency before prana moves up through the system.

There is believed to be an eighth chakra, *Asamprajnata Samadhi*. This chakra can be described as a condition where you are pure consciousness and nothing else. The activity of the mind is reset—you need nothing, know nothing but the present, and you feel free and united with everything around you. This is a kind of trance that can occur while doing yoga or meditation, as well as in your everyday life. Time stands still and one feels an enormous sense of happiness and peace in the soul. You forget time and place and are one with everything in the present.

Prana—what is it really?

Yoga is more than just movements. Yoga can be seen as a practical art form where bodily energy is released as you slowly develop these movements. This disengagement wakes up the inner life, and the possibility to receive and develop life power gets stronger. Life energy, or life power, is called *prana* in Sanskrit. It is an innate energy that human beings can always gain access to. It circulates in the body and creates life. It comes to us when we inhale, but it is more than just the oxygen we need to live.

According to the old sacred Hindu scriptures, prana is a vibrating psychophysical energy similar in nature to the concept of *pneuma*; an energy whose discussion dates to ancient Greece. Aristotle claims that the human being is an organism controlled by energy and that we are all part of a universal power that determines our physical and mental nature. Prana also bears comparison to the energy Albert Einstein refers to in his theory of relativity. Einstein claims that everything is a timeless flowing field of constant information, and the body is a flowing organism that has achieved its power through millions of years of intelligence. This intelligence, our mind, watches over the constant process of transformation that takes place in each and every one of us, and this intelligence affects each cell in the body.

Prana is the link between body, soul, matter, and energy. It is a universal power, a pure flow of energy that maintains the activity in your body, mind, and soul, while at the same time creating the movements in planets and stars. Prana is innate in all living things. This life power flows in our electromagnetic body through *nadis* (channels along, around, and through the spine), and it gives energy to all organs and cells in the body. Prana is a vitalizing power, and when you start practicing yoga, you learn consciously how to control and set prana into motion. This idea of a stream of life energy in the body can be also found in *qigong*, where the life power is called *qi*, or in Japanese martial arts, where life power is called *ki*. The chakras are stimulated when you perform different movements in yoga training. Tension and stress are reduced when the stream of energy induced by breathing starts flowing. This stream of energy can also be generated by the physical poses and *asanas*.

Power Yoga is focused on strength. You get stronger when you work with prana. The more prana you transport around inside the body, the more balanced, strong, and positive you get. It is hard to define prana precisely, but it is *not* just a mysterious power whose role it is to maintain equilibrium and to protect against imbalances and disturbances. Prana is a pure stream of energy that has an obvious purpose but doesn't resemble other limited mechanisms.

The first step to getting more prana in the body is to learn how to perform deep and conscious breathing. Breathing deeply promotes health, partially because it increases oxygen absorption and energy and partially because it leads to a higher degree of presence. By focusing on the present and your breathing, you can evaluate life and clamp down on "monkey mind"—the intense brain activity of a stressed-out mind.

[14] Chakra = 'wheel' or 'round disc' in Sanskrit.
[15] The wickerwork of nerves in the sacrum includes the ilioinguinalis nerve, which is connected to the muscles in the frontal lower part of the abdominal cavity and the skin on the genital organs.
[16] This gland is an important part of the immune defence. It is reduced after childhood.
[17] This is because of its relation to capaciousness and liberty of action.

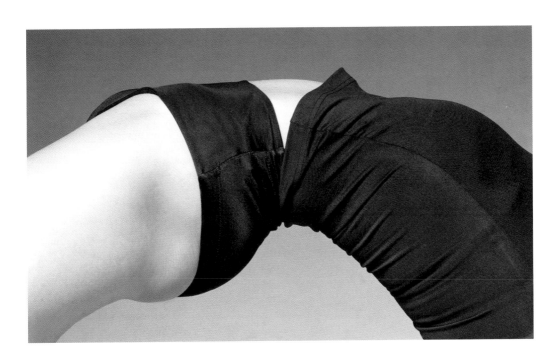

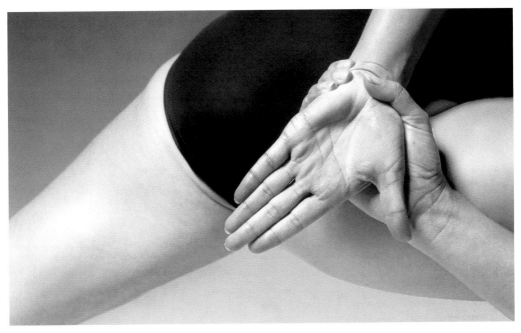

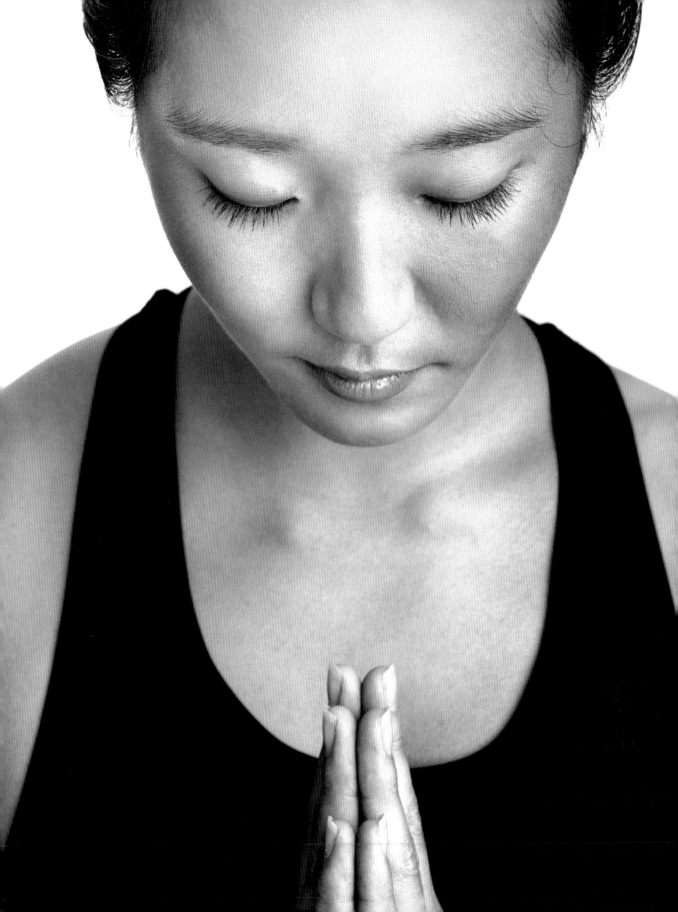

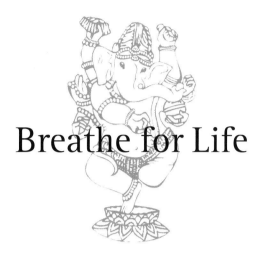

Breathe for Life

Breathing is like a thin thread that can become strong and powerful and be an excellent tool to help us handle situations that otherwise could seem impossible. Breathing is the bridge between our physical and our psychological self and the element that makes it possible for the body, the soul and the mind to become one unity. Breathing is like an engine that makes sure that we live, but conscious breathing can also make us stronger, more resistant, healthier, calmer and harmonic. — Thich Nhat Hanh

Great gurus in the yoga tradition believe we are born with a limited number of breaths. They claim that if we train our breath to be deeper and longer, we can prolong our life. Yoga tradition has always emphasized the importance of observing and controlling breath. In *Yoga Sutra* by Patanjali, *pranayama* (energy control; breathing) is described as one of the important paths to happiness, insight, power, and spiritual liberation. In Sanskrit, *prana* not only means breathing, it also means life power or life energy, the power that gives life to everything in the universe. *Yama* means control or "being able to master." Pranayama uses, trains, and strengthens the bodily respiration apparatus, but it is more than just inhalation and exhalation. Yogis and yoginis[18] use breathing to channel and absorb as much life power as possible in order to be able to use this power to promote and improve their personal evolution. They use breathing to make the body, soul, and mind stronger and to achieve a more harmonic life, one without physical and psychological limitations.

It is essential to learn breathing the right way if you want to be healthier and feel better. When you breathe, your lung capacity increases, the blood gets more oxygen, and that produces more life power, energizing your inner organs while at the same time cleansing them. Conscious and correct breathing also calms the nervous system. The deeper the breath, the calmer your mind feels. In yoga you concentrate on breathing using the diaphragm, and you always keep your mouth closed and breathe in and out through the nose. Breathing is not the same as inhaling air for life energy. The air is oxygen and is called *prana vajo* (vajo means "wind" in Sanskrit). The air you breathe sends the life energy (prana) through your body.

When you breathe consciously, the different parts of the body are influenced and start producing energy. This energy production is absorbed and taken in by the mind. Your breathing should be regular and flowing during the entire yoga training, regardless of whether or not you are bending forward, backwards, or to either side. When doing other physical activities, like running or aerobic exercises, a more mechanical kind of breathing is used. Here the frequency is increased, but it isn't very useful. Breathing is life—we breathe to live. Because of the increased absorption of oxygen into the cells and the balancing of the nervous system, conscious breathing makes you able to live *more* and be healthier.

Active exhalation

There are many different breathing techniques in yoga gathered under the term Paranayama; energy control or breathing control. To learn one of these techniques, you go through three steps. The first step is to train your diaphragm breathing (breathing with the stomach). This involves training the diaphragm to work harder and reduce the expansion of the chest. Here you focus on getting the diaphragm to work as well as possible in order to use your entire lung capacity. When breathing is optimized, waste products are eliminated and your circulation gets better. It also has a positive impact on the heart, liver, intestines, and other inner organs. A good way to establish a conscious and improved way of breathing is to start using *active exhalation*. This technique is the direct opposite of unconscious breathing, in which you breathe in and out in a passive way, and helps healing prana flow into tense muscles, injured areas, and the inner organs. Active exhalation makes you feel in contact with the diaphragm's breathing muscle, and it activates the area around the *solar plexus*[19], the midriff. This is especially helpful if you want to master the *Ujjayi Pranayama*, the primary breathing technique utilized in Power Yoga.

Seat yourself in the pose *Padmasana* (page 62), sit cross-legged, kneel, or stand up in *Tadasana* (page 61).

1. Place one hand on your solar plexus and the other on the lower part of the stomach. Close your mouth.

2. Focus on your exhalation. Inhale with your mouth closed and concentrate on letting the lower part of your chest move downwards at the same time as you contract (tighten) the muscles in your stomach, so that the stomach moves towards the spine and the diaphragm is lifted.

3. Repeat this several times. Focus on the exhalation. Slowly press out all the air. Stop. Let go in your chest and stomach. Keep your mouth closed when you inhale and exhale. Yoga breathing always happens through the nose (avoid "snorting" when you exhale, but keep the nostrils relaxed).

4. If it doesn't work, then just let the inhalation "happen" by relaxing after each exhale and hold your breath for a few seconds. Don't try to inhale. When you have learned the technique, you will feel the diaphragm moving towards the chest when you exhale and lowering when you inhale. After practicing this type of breathing for a period of time (start by using it in yoga training and move on to step 5 when you feel ready), you will learn how to breathe the right way. The process of focusing and listening to your breathing will then become easier and soon feel natural to you. Active exhalation is a great technique that develops your breathing, making it stronger and more effective. It also makes you more conscious of the positive effects of breathing. Active exhalation gives you peace of mind and makes you concentrate better.

5. When you feel ready to move on, you can start alternating your breathing exercises. Calmly press out the exhalation *and* inhale actively. Make each breath last longer. Now try to keep the sound of your breathing "in the middle of your head" and listen to it. Try to seat yourself in the Half Lotus Pose. Finally, you can replace this breathing technique with the more complicated *Ujjayi*-breathing (page 48). Abdominal breathing has a very positive effect: it calms the mind and helps the circulation (it also burns calories). It makes it easier to concentrate and it eliminates waste products. At the same time it is very useful for the inner organs, supplying them with energy and the "oil" they need to perform.

Training the diaphragm

The diaphragm is a thin fan-shaped membrane, located in front of the spine between the chest and the stomach. Seen from below it looks like the sky, and seen from above it looks like a hill. It supplies all the stomach organs with "nerve energy." When you breathe the right way, the organs in the stomach are massaged. The diaphragm is lowered, and it massages the liver so that more blood runs to it. The blood is pressed out during exhalation. When you exhale, the transverse abdominal muscles are activated as well as the muscles below the ribs, pressing out any residual air[20]. If you breathe the wrong way, the nerve cells, whose job it is to generate and lead the different electrochemical types of energy called nerve impulses, don't get completely recharged.

Ujjayi-breathing. After practicing yoga for a while, you might feel it's time to develop your breathing even further. The next step after active breathing is *Ujjayi Pranayama. Uj* means "to expand," or "widen"; *jayi* means "gain, elevate." It is important to understand that breathing develops and changes when you start doing yoga. At the beginning, you can't master the more difficult breathing techniques, just as you can't do the more advanced yoga poses and movements. It might take months or years before it feels right to move on to the next level (and getting to the next level may not be yoga's purpose in your life). Go at a pace that feels right to you.

Learning Ujjayi-breathing is learning the very language of Power Yoga. In the same way an actor practices his lines or a dancer learns new steps, you train your conscious breathing to ultimately achieve a level of perfection. In short, you can control your mind when you control your breathing. If you want to control something like water, traffic, or breathing, you must narrow the passage that the energy of life flows through. To get water into your faucet, the water must be lead from a lake or from the waterworks into a pipe. Breathing control works the same way. When you consciously narrow the passage in the throat where the air passes through, you can prolong your breathing and in that way control it.

Ujjayi-breathing makes a specific roaring sound when the air is led over the larynx and the vocal chords. The same goes for whispering. The contraction in the throat when you inhale and exhale increases the speed of the air that is passing and reduces the air passage. That is what makes the roaring sound. You can compare the Ujjayi-sound to the sound of a sea breeze or the way Darth Vader in *Star Wars* breathes. Even though Ujjayi-breathing is done through the nose and with your mouth closed, it is easier to learn this kind of breathing with your mouth opened.

1. Start whispering an "ah" or an "uh" sound with your mouth opened when you exhale. Try to empty the air in your lungs using the sound.

2. Inhale again while whispering "ah" or "uh." Fill the lungs with air. Focus on your stomach (the diaphragm).

3. Do the same with your mouth closed. The inhalation will create a howling sound, and the exhalation will make a hissing sound—as if you were trying to whisper with your mouth closed. When you inhale, you must imagine that you are "pulling" your breath from the bottom of your spine up towards the diaphragm from where you calmly exhale. Let the stomach dilate when you inhale and contract when you exhale. Listen to the breathing and keep the sound in the middle of your head, behind the neck.

4. If you start coughing or feeling badly when practicing Ujjayi-breathing, it is because you're trying too hard. The elimination of waste products is speeded up too quickly (don't worry—this isn't dangerous). Practice this kind of breathing slowly. Keep your mouth closed and breathe through your nose. Try placing one hand on your stomach and the other on your diaphragm. Close your eyes and feel yourself breathing. Don't give up even if it doesn't work the first several times. Train yourself until it becomes routine. If you still think it is difficult, take a step back and try again at some other time.

Ujjayi-breathing, when it's done optimally, generates heat and helps you concentrate and focus during meditation or any time you feel stressed out. It also eases your mind when asking your body to perform hard physical work (for example, during childbirth). The power of correct, conscious breathing is enormous. It can ease illnesses, give you healthier skin, reduce the nuisances that come with smoking or sugar, and relieve depression and aggression, as well as give you a higher appreciation of life.

Ujjayi-breathing, described in *Yoga Korunta*, is one of the secret Indian techniques that has been passed on to Western yoga performers who studied yoga under the Indian yoga masters. Combined with yoga training, the Ujjayi-breathing is a perfect tool to even out bodily imbalances, achieve strength, get better balance, flexibility, and mobility, as well as to emancipate the body and the inner organs from impurities and poisonous substances. Conscious breathing and asanas also clear the mind and strengthen the soul in the present. Movement and breathing can't be separated! When you breathe in the "right" way, the diaphragm is trained, and your lung capacity and level of performance improve. When you feel that you have mastered Ujjayi-breathing during as well as after yoga training, you can—if you want to—go a step further and integrate the so called "body locks," or *bandhas*. A body lock is a muscular contraction that is used to focus your concentration, stimulate heat, and control prana—the psychosomatic energy called life power. Bandhas is a complicated training of the muscles and it can take years to get it right. There are two different body locks that are parts of Power Yoga's more advanced sequences.

Mula Bandha — Root Lock. When you do a Root Lock you tighten and lift the perineum muscle[21] — the perineum muscle that is placed between the genital organs and anus. First the perineum muscle is lifted up and tightened. After that you inhale and let the stomach dilate.

Uddiyana Bandha — Stomach Lock. When you do the Stomach Lock, you either lead the navel away from or towards the spine. This activates all the muscular groups in the stomach. Exhale and pull your stomach inwards and up towards the chest using your stomach muscles at the same time as you are pressing the lower part of the chest towards the spine. Inhale and repeat the exercise.

Do these two different kinds of body locks during the same breathing routine. Tighten the perineum muscle (Root Lock) and inhale. Exhale and activate the Stomach Lock.

[18] *Yogi = male yoga practitioner. Yogini = female yoga practitioner.*

[19] *The solar plexus is the area between the chest and the stomach. The word solar fits well for this area since the abdominal "brain" in the abdominal cavity radiates strength and energy. Plexus (Latin: a bundle of nerves; here: accumulation of nerves and ganglions, nerve fibers) are coupling stations along the spine and storage room for the energy of the nervous system. According to yoga teachings, this center is a huge storage room for prana, and in both the East and West it's seen as the center of emotional expression.*

[20] *Residual air is the air that always stays in the lungs.*

[21] *It can be hard to find this muscle. Women: start by tightening the vaginal muscles — and men: tighten the ring muscle/sphincter. This activates the perineum muscle. After a lot of training, you'll be able to find and tighten the perineum muscle automatically.*

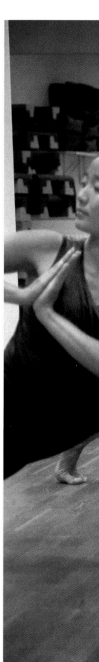

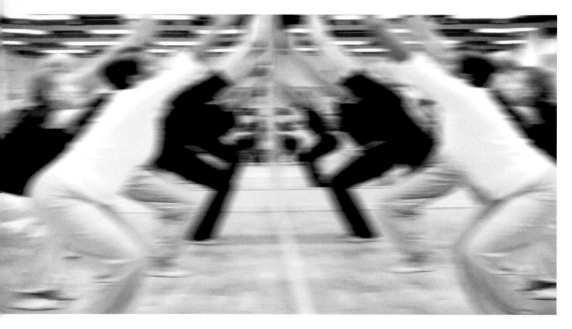

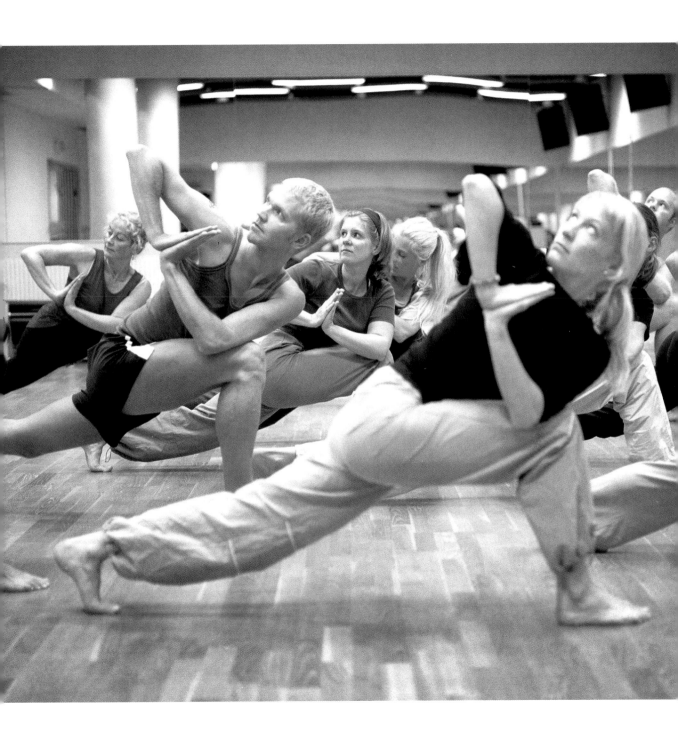

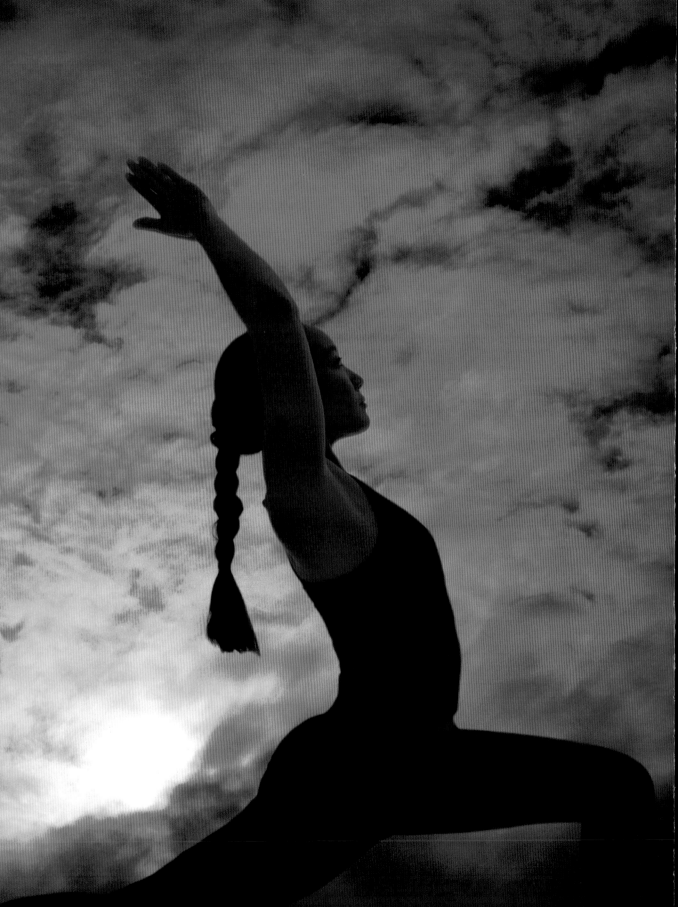

Salute the Sun

Sun salutation is a complete sequence of movements that warm up the muscles and joints, the starting point for Power Yoga training. In Sanskrit, Sun Salutation is called *Surya Mamaskar*, which means "graceful, beloved salute to the sun." There are two different kinds of Sun Salutations in Power Yoga. Sun Salutation A has nine poses (the modified version has more), and Sun Salutation B has seventeen poses. Both of the Sun Salutations generate heat, help you to focus, are physically dynamic, and take place in one flowing movement. The spine is the structural core in Power Yoga, and the Sun Salutation makes your physical and mental awareness of the spine stronger.

Many of us suffer from imbalances in the body. They stem from bad posture, different kinds of injuries, one-sided training, or sedentary work. When we move through the poses in the Sun Salutation, the muscles get stronger and warmer along the spine. This focus and concentrated breathing makes us aware of how mobility gets limited over the years. The Sun Salutation generates a lot of heat in the body on all levels and at the same time softens and develops the natural flexibility of the spine. If you analyze each single step in these movements, you will find that, together, the different elements are the basis of the dynamical structure of the Sun Salutation. You stretch yourself upwards and downwards. You stretch yourself forwards and backwards. You carry your entire weight on your upper body. You carry your entire weight on your lower body. You contract the muscles on both the back and front sides of the body. You expand the muscles on both the back and front sides of the body. Contraction and expansion are the basis of the strong and soft elements in Power Yoga. You start working on one muscle and then let it rest. This is repeated over and over again during the entire yoga training. The neuro-muscular system finds a natural balance between these two elementary conditions. The Sun Salutation is the beginning of the bodily process that is the purpose of Power Yoga: to contract and stretch out not only each single muscle, but also to stretch one muscle at the same time as you are contracting another. The muscle work takes place simultaneously.

Warm muscles reduce imbalances

Nothing can make your muscles and joints more thoroughly warm than the Sun Salutation. Light jogging, aerobic work, and biking on an exercise bike warm up the legs and activate the cardiovascular system, but what about arms, shoulders, and spine? Aerobic exercise warms you up, but it doesn't mediate the combination of rest and activity in the muscles. The Sun Salutation warms up the joints and the muscular tissue using the right frequency of softening movements. Many people begin physical activity with stretching exercises, but that's not the same as warming up. To increase the mobility in muscles and joints, you must be warm and not have too high a pulse. Heat means heat from working the muscles inside out and not heat from taking a hot bath or shower! If the body is cold when you do stretching exercises, stretching has almost no effect, and you risk injuries. Stretching out after aerobics is far safer but not very efficient, because the body is cooling down. Doing Power Yoga speeds up this process. Many people are astonished that they get so warm and that their mobility gets so much better after doing Power Yoga only two or three times! The uniqueness of yoga is that you only stretch out the muscles while the body is warm.

It's too big a job to learn all the elements of yoga all at once. *"How on earth am I going to think about breathing, bandhas—whatever that might be—and work hard and stay focused while I'm trying to remember all the movements?"* The elements[22] in yoga training can be compared to streams that each run on their own but finally run together at the mouth of a river before streaming into an ocean. Try working on the elements one by one until you're familiar with them all. Take one step at a time.

The meaning of the sun in ancient India

The sun was central in human life and thought in ancient India. Every morning the sun was worshipped. The sun was the symbol of the great light and the pure insight that people hoped to find in themselves. Traditionally, you closed your eyes just after having seen the morning sun in the hope of finding the same light and strength in yourself. The golden sun was the guiding symbol of the divine. To the Indians, the sun was the god above all gods. It was claimed that everything positive came from the sun and that the higher energies gave positive power to the human beings on Earth. They believed that this positive power created hope and faith and gave them the strength to be able to handle life on earth. The gold color on Buddha and Krishna figurines represents the divine because these two both possessed great wisdom and insight. The sun generates heat, and yogis claim that if you close your eyes during the Sun Salutation, your thoughts are guided to the golden ball, creating even more strength and energy. The Sun Salutation warms up all the cells in your body and nourishes them with oxygen. The heat generated in the Sun Salutation eliminates poisonous substances and impurities in the muscles, organs, skin, mind, and soul.

The importance of breathing

A lot of people feel tension in their muscles even though they regularly exercise, be it running, biking, dancing, strength training, or even badminton. Many of us who work out find that exercise is an opportunity to let go of thoughts concerning our jobs, or any demands and obligations that we have, and get the energy to do other things. You feel refreshed and stronger, even though our stress might still be there. Power Yoga is based on the principle that changes in your consciousness can only take place if we wake up our inner energy and allow it to flow. The first step on the journey is to turn the body into a healthy, mobile, and controlled tool for the powers that are in us. Yet mobility and physical training alone don't get these inner streams flowing or activate our inner strength. It is *breathing* that unites the body with the consciousness. *Hatha Yoga Pradipika* by Swami Svatmarama is one of the classical texts about yoga. In it, he writes that the mind (in this case the brain) is believed to be the god of the body, and *prana* is the god of the mind. Since prana is taken in through breathing, you will soon sense that breathing works like a bridge between movement and consciousness. When your breathing gets stronger and you succeed in focusing on it, the awareness of your body increases. That also means that your sense of the right posture and balance in the poses becomes better. You achieve a higher ability to develop your yoga training. When the breathing develops and becomes stronger and more powerful, the movements are easier to do, the muscles get warmer and softer, and you feel the mind calming down. Harmony comes to you. Everything in you starts operating on the same frequency, and this is the place where you can achieve true well-being. You feel strong, focused, and calm; no other thoughts can disturb you in your training. Your body is grateful for the energy that you have given to it and you feel amazing afterwards.

Flexibility is not the goal!

While working with this book, you might think: "*No way will I ever be able to do that pose.*" And you're right; you might not be able to do it . . . right now. However, you may be able to do it in a couple of weeks. Try it first. Some poses you won't be able to do for years. Don't be scared away by the pictures. Just read the text beneath each picture and try to perform the movement as the text describes it according to your own abilities. Pay attention to how far you can go. You should not aim for flexibility. That will only frustrate you.

Many beginners that train in my classes progress quickly. I myself was extremely tense in the muscles around my shoulders and hips and the front and back sides of my thighs when I started doing yoga nine years ago. One-sided work positions, injuries from skiing, basketball, volleyball, dancing, biking, and excessive aerobic exercise had made my muscles tense around the joints, and there were constant signs of imbalance. On top of that, I had digestive problems and was prone to catching colds. When I started doing yoga, I tried to copy the yoga instructor's movements, but that only led to frustration because I couldn't meet my own expectations of being able to execute the perfect pose. Yet when I let go of those thoughts, I felt much better. Today, many years and a lot of yoga lessons later, my digestive problems have almost disappeared. After a yoga session, I very seldom feel stiffness in my muscles, and I'm hardly ever ill anymore.

How do I start?

Spend some time on this chapter and pay attention to each pose in the Sun Salutation. The Sun Salutation sequence is built by performing smaller sequences, and poor technique at the beginning will haunt you later on. Aim at getting the right posture in your body when you do the movements. Don't think about how it looks but about how it feels. Listen to your body and read the instructions carefully! Work *with* the body, not against it. Feel them but don't stress yourself out in order to get balance. In many of the poses described in the following chapter, the effects of the exercises are explained. These can be achieved if you train regularly. Once a week is enough, and you don't have to do all the exercises. The most important thing is that you always do an initial exercise (Sun Salutation A & B), a middle exercise (standing and seated poses), and a final exercise (relaxation/mental relaxation).

Preparations: Make sure that there is peace around you when you do yoga and choose a harmonious place with natural lighting. Use a yoga mat if you have one. Lower the light if possible. Light a candle perhaps and put on quiet and pleasant music. Disconnect the phone. If your sense of time isn't good, use a timer.

Sit down with your legs crossed *(Half Lotus Pose)* and keep your back straight. Relax your shoulders and arms. Close your eyes and start deep breathing and active exhalation. Try concentrating on breathing down towards the diaphragm, and keep your back straight. Continue until you feel more at ease and in touch with your body. When you close your eyes, you only have to concentrate on your breathing, but if thoughts are running around in your head, try to focus on a color—white, yellow, or red—and push the thoughts away. If you still feel stressed, you can massage yourself (head, shoulders, and face) or lie down on your back for a while and try to relax.

1. Don't stress yourself when you enter into a yoga movement. Always follow the instructions! Let the movements be soft and calm and avoid sudden movements in the body. Immediately stop the movement if you feel pain in your muscles or joints. Don't put pressure on yourself, and always do the exercises according to your own abilities. Pay attention to your posture. Remember that yoga isn't a competitive sport, and if you do yoga with someone who's more experienced than you, you should not compare yourself to him or her and be

tempted to try and reach the same level in the poses. Find your own level of development. Concentrate on listening to your breathing, relax the mind, and focus on the present.

2. Yoga prescribes cleanliness. People who do yoga speed up inner as well as outer cleansing processes. According to classical yoga literature, you should shower, wash your feet, and cut your nails before doing yoga. Strange body odors might occur while doing yoga. That's because poisonous substances and waste products are leaving the body. It takes about 3 to 6 weeks before the body odor disappears completely.

3. Be aware of how far you can enter into the movements and listen to your body every time you breathe. Your physical sensations are your body's voice and therefore your guide to your own safety! Make sure the floor is clean and without objects that can distract you. Do the exercises with bare feet.

4. It is good to train in the morning when you set the foundation for the entire day. If you do 20 minutes of yoga before breakfast, the body is supplied with energy, the metabolism gets stronger, and you can focus better on your workday.

5. If you are menstruating, you should pay attention to what feels good and bad. It is not dangerous to do yoga during your period, but certain exercises might feel unpleasant. If that is the case, don't do them! I've had no problems myself and actually feel better if I do yoga during my period. In general, you should skip inverted poses during the heavy days or just take a break from physical yoga for 2 to 3 days. It is good to focus on breathing and meditate instead. Are you pregnant? Congratulations! Generally speaking you should be able to feel what you can or cannot do. Usually there are no problems in doing Power Yoga for the first 3 to 4 months of your pregnancy IF you are an experienced yogini. After that, you should ask your yoga teacher to give you alternative exercises. Find special programs for pregnant women, or find a school that gives classes to pregnant women, or train at home using a plan that has been made by your yoga teacher.

6. Drink a lot of water before and after the training. Dehydration can create imbalances and illnesses. Avoid drinking during the actual training and for 20 to 30 minutes after it. This is the period where the cleansing of the inner organs takes place (liver, intestines, kidneys, etc). Fluid in the intestines "disturbs" the process. Avoid doing yoga just after eating. Wait for 3 to 4 hours after a big meal or an hour after a snack. If you do this, your mental focus and breathing will get stronger, and your metabolism gets better after training. It might feel unpleasant and lead to irritation, dizziness, and indisposition

to train with food in your stomach. This happens because the many movements and exercises you perform may increase the intra-abdominal pressure and affect the inner organs.

7. Be careful with relaxation after the Sun Salutation, as well as the standing and seated asanas. The body has to relax when it returns to its normal state so you can experience the positive effects from the exercise. Never leave out the last exercise, Corpse Pose. The longer the relaxation period is (preferably 7 to 10 minutes), the deeper you relax, and from that your nervous system gets relaxed. No matter when you do yoga, remember the basic facts: body and mind should control the movements; follow the rhythm of the breathing; do the movements slowly; and concentrate on your breathing, as well as on how your body feels. You can try leading your conscious breathing towards the area where the muscles are stretched. It is also very important to push away the idea of performance and results when you do the exercise. Answer any thought with a breath and avoid holding on to the thought. Just focus on the present moment and how your body feels.

Different movements fit different people. If you feel an exercise is hard to do, you can modify it until it feels easier. Also, don't focus on just one area of your body. Yoga is all about balancing the body, and you can't do that if you become flexible only in one area. That will only make the stiffness somewhere else in your body worse. We are all unique individuals with different bodies, and we're not intended to do the movements in the same ways. Respect your body and its qualifications. Then you will achieve balance quicker!

8. Reverse poses should be avoided (or in some cases modified) if you suffer from high blood pressure, ear problems, decompression sickness, back pains, illnesses, dizziness, obesity, glaucoma, or if you have eye problems. If you have recently undergone surgery, you should talk to your doctor. Besides that, almost anyone, no matter his or her age, can do yoga!

Asanas

One of the basic elements in yoga training is to maintain a good posture in seated as well as standing poses, and many of the exercises have been developed in order to stretch the muscles in their length. This enables you to keep your back straight. Whether or not you are standing or sitting on your knees, you should imagine that there is a string that pulls the head towards the ceiling. "Open" your chest by pulling your shoulder blades together. Then the chest has a natural lift.

You can start the training in two ways

1. One way is to start in a standing pose, *Tadasana*, and take eight deep breaths. After this, inhale. When you exhale, slowly let yourself fall forward, keeping your legs as straight as possible in *Head to Knee Pose.* Keep standing like this and find your balance on your heels. Keep the feet at shoulders' width. Relax the shoulders, neck, face, and arms. Close your eyes and take at least eight deep breaths. This pose is also called *Resting Head to Knee.*

From here, you start *Sun Salutation* A by inhaling and straightening your back. Let your arms hang down in front of you and look straight down. Bend your knees a little and keep the back tightened. Exhale. Inhale and slowly lift your eyes towards the ceiling while still keeping a straight back. Lead the arms upwards/outwards and exhale. If your back hurts, you can bend your knees a little. If you're a beginner, you can roll up slowly in your back and focus on the floor. Keep your stomach tightened and relax the arms, shoulders, and neck.

2. The second, more common way, to start yoga training begins with the *Lotus Pose.* Here you breathe with your eyes closed for a couple of minutes. The pose is followed by *Tolasana* A, *Tolasana* B (pages 62–63), and finally *Resting Head to Knee.* The transition to *Sun Salutation* A is then done in the same way as mentioned above.

Surya Namaskara A: Sun Salutation A

This sequence of poses or asanas is the introduction to yoga training. It increases body heat, concentration, and focus. To learn this sequence of asanas (pages 64–71), you must do one pose at a time and hold it while you take five breaths in order to feel the pose properly. When you've been through all the movements, they can be linked together into one flowing movement. Use your breathing as the engine that keeps you going. If you get tired and your pulse raises, you can rest by taking a few deep breaths in *the Child Pose* (page 99).

[22] *Power Yoga has five elements: Ujjayi-breathing, concentration, static muscular contraction, vinyasa, and bandhas.*

Tadasana: the Mountain Pose

Tadasana is the basic pose in yoga.

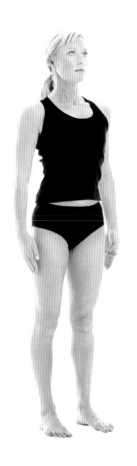 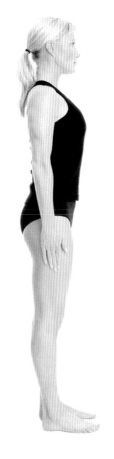 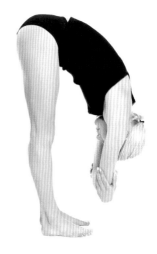

Resting Head to Knee: Bend over forward keeping your legs as straight as possible. Stay here and find the balance on the heels. Keep the feet at shoulders' width and hold elbows with your hands. Relax your shoulders, neck, face, and arms.

Tadasana is a dynamic pose where you should concentrate on each single muscle in the body. Stand with your legs spread (feet at shoulders' width, knees slightly bent if you are a beginner or if you have back problems). Put the main weight on your heels. That helps you keep an even balance on the entire sole of the foot. Relax your shoulders, roll them backwards and tighten the shoulder blade muscles a little. Let the arms hang down at the sides of your body. Push the pelvis forward slightly so that the stomach is tightened and the spine is straight. Tighten the front side of the thighs. Focus on the floor in front of you. Don't sway, but if you do, bend your knees a little and tighten the stomach.

Lotus Padmasana

Begins with Tadasana and is followed by the Lotus Lift and the Turtle Lift.

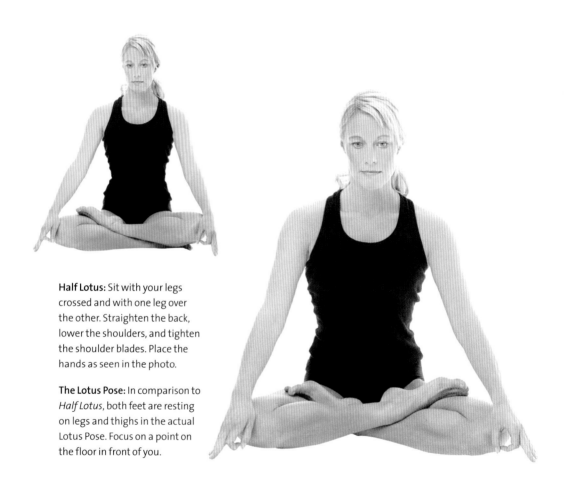

Half Lotus: Sit with your legs crossed and with one leg over the other. Straighten the back, lower the shoulders, and tighten the shoulder blades. Place the hands as seen in the photo.

The Lotus Pose: In comparison to *Half Lotus*, both feet are resting on legs and thighs in the actual Lotus Pose. Focus on a point on the floor in front of you.

The Lotus Pose is demanding and can be hard for beginners. Wait until you are more flexible in the knees, feet, and hip joints. Concentrate on sitting comfortably in *Half Lotus* instead and focus on your breathing. The most important thing is to push the base of the pelvis into the floor and to keep a straight back. If *Half Lotus* is too difficult, you can sit on your knees, put your hands in your lap, and breathe. If you have a hard time collecting your thoughts, close your eyes and concentrate on the color red.

This pose centers your balance and gives you a positive feeling.

Tolasana A: Lotus Lift

Begins with Lotus Padmasana and is followed by the Turtle Lift.

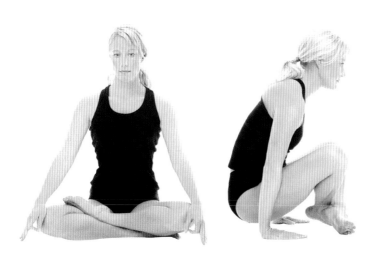

1. Be seated in *Half Lotus* (advanced: be seated in the *Lotus Pose*). Place your hands or your knuckles next to your buttocks and stretch the fingers forward. Inhale and look at your legs.

2. Exhale and lift your buttocks and legs from the floor using the hands. Tighten the shoulders, back, and stomach and lift the knees towards the shoulders. Look in at the body. Try moving the head away from the shoulders. Take four deep breaths and put the emphasis on exhalation. Lower yourself when you exhale for the last time.

Tolasana B: Diamond Lift

Begins with Tolasana A and is followed by Sun Salutation A.

1. Sit on your knees with your legs gathered. Place the hands (or the knuckles) next to the knees and stretch your fingers forwards. Inhale.

2. Exhale. Lift the knees towards the chest and keep the top sides of the feet on the floor. Move the shoulders away and look inwards at the body. Take four deep breaths and put the emphasis on exhalation. Lower yourself to your knees when exhaling the last time.

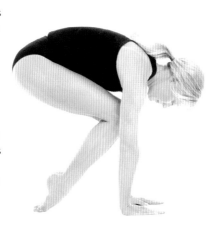

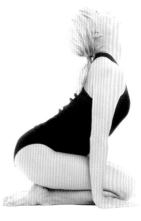

3. Inhale, point out the chest, tighten the back muscles, and look backwards. Exhale and repeat step 2.

Surya Namaskara A: Sun Salutation A

Is shown in sequences. On the following pages the movements are singled out.

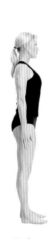

1. Tadasana

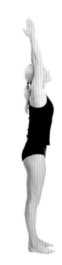

2. Sama-sthiti

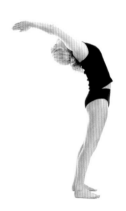

3. Sama-sthiti—Back Bend

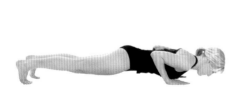

7. The Plank Position

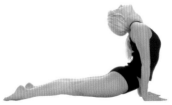

8. Upward Facing Dog

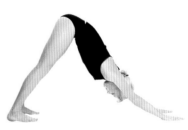

9. Downward Facing Dog

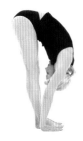

4. Head to Knee

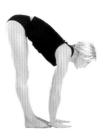

5. Look up

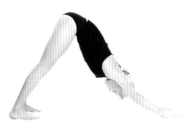

6. Downward Facing Dog

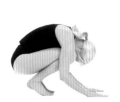

10. Squatting Pose

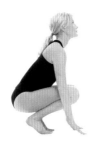

11. Squatting Pose—Look up

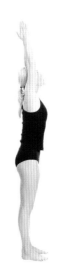

12. Sama-sthiti

Sama-sthiti: Concentration

Begins with Tadasana and is followed by Uttanasana.

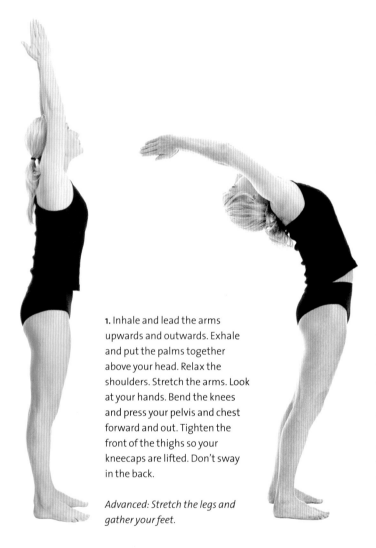

2. Lift the body as high as you can to make the body longer and pull up the chest. Exhale and relax the shoulders. Keep on stretching the arms above your head. Tighten the stomach.

1. Inhale and lead the arms upwards and outwards. Exhale and put the palms together above your head. Relax the shoulders. Stretch the arms. Look at your hands. Bend the knees and press your pelvis and chest forward and out. Tighten the front of the thighs so your kneecaps are lifted. Don't sway in the back.

Advanced: Stretch the legs and gather your feet.

3. Inhale and bend your knees, press the pelvis forward, tighten the stomach, and let the arms fall backwards. Look at a point on the ceiling. Don't drop your back or your arms.

Advanced: Follow the hands backwards with the eyes. Keep the shoulders relaxed, tighten the stomach, and keep the arms stretched.

A tightened muscle without a following movement is called a *static contraction*, and it signifies the "hard" sun aspect in Power Yoga. Static contraction uses energy and demands fuel, but it creates heat and keeps perspiration going. This muscular work is an essential part of the training and one of the five basic components of Power Yoga.

Uttanasana: Head to Knee

Begins with Sama-sthiti and is followed by Downward Facing Dog.

1. From the last pose: exhale, bend over, and place the arms in front of the stretched legs. Look at the floor. Keep a straight back all the way through this exercise. Tighten the front side of the thighs if your legs are stretched. The entire soles of your feet should rest on the floor. Imagine that someone is pulling your buttocks backwards using a string.

If it is hard to keep your legs stretched, then bend the knees a little but keep an even balance on both legs.

2. Place your hands (or bend the knees a little and place your fingertips) on the floor in front of the feet. Relax in neck and shoulders. Look in at the body. Don't force the body forward.

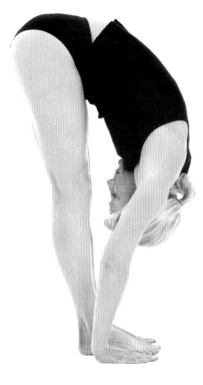

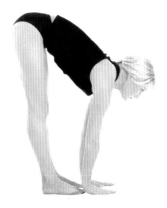

3. Look up. Inhale at the same time as you stretch the back, shoot out the chest, and look at the floor in front of you. Don't bend in the back. Keep it as straight as possible. Exhale and look at your legs.

Advanced: Try keeping the legs stretched. Tighten the muscles on the front side of the thighs.

When you're able to control your breathing, you will experience the joy and the positive effect in deep stretching exercises. You might feel a little stiff on the back of your thighs and across the loin. If you get a little dizzy, you should straighten out the back slowly and/or put your hands on a wall for a while. Keep the legs stretched and the back straight. Slow down and take one step at a time. After you have trained with Power Yoga regularly, you can try to proceed to the next step. It is important not to advance too quickly but to work with your body to ready it for the next step.

In this pose, the spine is made longer in a natural way, and it is a fantastic exercise to increase flexibility on the back side of the body. At the same time, it eliminates poisonous substances from the muscles and the bodily organs. Additionally, the brain and the nervous system are relaxed and balanced.

Adho Mukha Svanasana: Downward Facing Dog

Begins with Head to Knee and Look Up and is followed by the Plank Position.

1. Inhale and walk backwards until the body is standing like a pyramid, hands and feet at shoulders' width. Try to keep the legs stretched. Look inwards at your stomach.

2. Exhale and look at your feet. Shoot the body weight from the hands down towards the heels. Let the body "fall" through the arms. Lift the coccyx towards the ceiling and lead the stomach towards the front side of the thighs. Tighten the thighs and straighten the back.

If you have back problems, try bending the legs a little, but keep on pressing the heels in the floor. If you are stiffer in one side than the other, you should avoid bending only one leg. Keep an even balance.

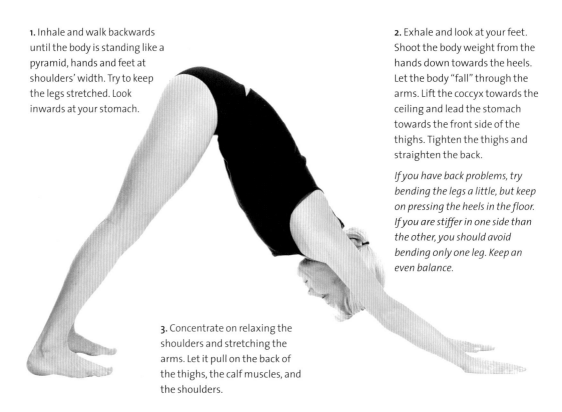

3. Concentrate on relaxing the shoulders and stretching the arms. Let it pull on the back of the thighs, the calf muscles, and the shoulders.

Spread your fingers so the palm has full contact with the floor. Place the weight on the lower part of the palm. To avoid tension in the shoulders, try "dropping" the shoulders, and relax your neck. When you stand in this pose for the first time, you should keep it for a while and just breathe. Try closing your eyes. Make sure that the feet are parallel. It is important that the heels don't point outwards when you lower yourself. This will happen without you knowing it because the body tries to avoid the pull on the back side of the thighs. Don't worry if you can't get your heels to touch the floor! It might take some time to get the heels all the way down without problems.

This pose stretches the entire body. Not only does this increase blood circulation, it also strengthens and brings out the muscles in legs, arms, stomach, and shoulders, prevents fatigue, and brings vitality both to bodily organs and muscles.

Chaturanga Dandasana: the Plank Position

Begins with Downward Facing Dog and is followed by Upward Facing Dog.

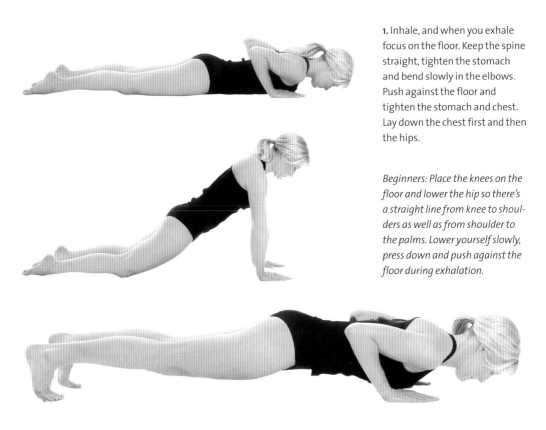

1. Inhale, and when you exhale focus on the floor. Keep the spine straight, tighten the stomach and bend slowly in the elbows. Push against the floor and tighten the stomach and chest. Lay down the chest first and then the hips.

Beginners: Place the knees on the floor and lower the hip so there's a straight line from knee to shoulders as well as from shoulder to the palms. Lower yourself slowly, press down and push against the floor during exhalation.

2. When you feel stronger, you can try to push yourself all the way down using the arms. Keep your eyes focused on the floor and keep the body horizontally stretched. Tighten the entire body and keep it above the floor.

Advanced: Keep yourself a little above the mat. Tighten the body. Tighten the legs, back, and stomach. Avoid rolling down. If it gets too hard, you can move the hands a little.

It is important that you tighten your back and your stomach, focus on the floor, and avoid the elbows pointing to both sides. To not put strain on the shoulders, you must let the chest meet the floor before the hip.

This pose works and strengthens the back, stomach, chest, and seat. It also increases life power in the intestines, liver, and kidneys.

Urdhva Mukha Svanasana: Upward Facing Dog

Begins with the Plank Position and is followed by the Plank Position and Downward Facing Dog.

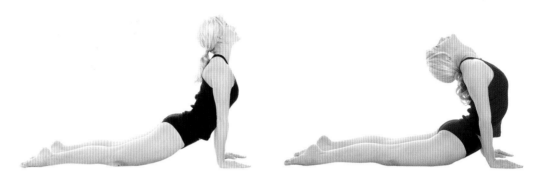

1. Inhale and look upwards/backwards. Push away from the floor with your hands and shoot the chest forward. Turn the soles of your feet towards the ceiling. With your shoulders back, tighten the shoulder blades and avoid "hanging" in the shoulders. Tighten the arms.

Beginners: Keep your knees on the floor and bend the back as far backwards as you can.

2. Exhale, focus on the floor and return to the Plank Position (page 69). Tighten the arms and the stomach and push against them. Don't drop the back. Return back to *Downward Facing Dog* (page 68).

Advanced: do a Toe Roll and move to the top side of the foot.

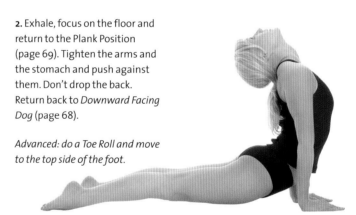

The Toe Roll is hard to do if the muscles and foot joints are tight. Avoid performing the toe roll until your flexibility has increased. This pose can cause soreness in the loin area if you do it the wrong way. Try to avoid swaying or hanging in the shoulders. If you have back problems, let the knees stay on the floor in all *Dog Poses*. Push your head away from the shoulders and shoot the chest forward. Tighten the stomach—and look backwards! It is also important that the entire palm touches the floor and that the arms are engaged.

In this exercise the back muscles get strong and shaped, especially the lower part of the back. It also gives you firmer buttocks, and it heightens the intra-abdominal pressure that balances and strengthens the uterus and the ovaries. At the same time, it improves your intestinal functions. Also, the menstrual cycle is regulated, and the thyroid gland works more efficiently.

Squatting Pose

Begins with Downward Facing Dog and is followed by Sama-sthiti.

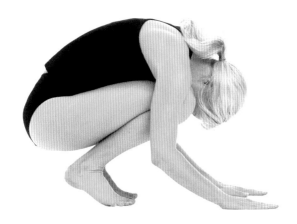

1. From *Downward Facing Dog:* Look at your feet. Inhale, bend the knees, and exhale at the same time as walking or hopping forwards into *the Squatting Pose.*

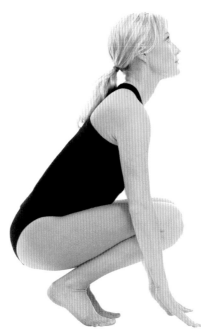

For beginners or if you have knee or back problems: Seat yourself with your feet at shoulders' width.

2. Inhale, look at the ceiling, straighten the back, and lead the arms upwards and outwards. Exhale and slowly push away from the floor, letting the arms move towards the ceiling. Avoid rolling into standing position.

The Squatting Pose is an added pose for beginners in the Sun Salutation. It is discarded when the strength of the spine is more in balance. The pose is followed by *Sama-sthiti*, which is used as a link between the *Sun Salutation* A and the next sequence. Stay in the pose while taking a couple of breaths. Return and repeat the sequence (pages 64–65). Try doing four to eight *Sun Salutation* A's before moving on to *Sun Salutation B.*

WARNING

You maintain your heat when you maintain your concentration during all the exercises in the Sun Salutation. If you lose concentration in yoga, you will feel the heat dissipating. It takes concentration to keep the static contraction in the muscles at the same time as keeping your breath going. Try doing between four and eight *Sun Salutation* A sequences, one after another.

If a problem occurs during the exercises, you can do the simpler versions as described. If you have an injury and want to start doing yoga, you must start slowly—even if you're an elite athlete, dancer, or just very fit. Yoga will help you through the regeneration phase.

Possible side effects in Sun Salutation

Many people have limited mobility because of injuries, stiff muscles and joints, and weaknesses in certain parts of their body. If you're new to yoga, watch for these warning signs:

It hurts in the shoulders. If this happens when you enter into and out of the *Dog Pose*, it is because you are "hanging" in the shoulders in *Upward Facing Dog*. This might happen because the muscles in the upper body are weak. You therefore compensate by overstretching the shoulders when you enter the *Plank Position*. That isn't good for the back and the shoulders. Try to use the modified examples instead. If that hurts your arms, you may have overstretched them. Try to tighten them all the time in the *Dog Pose* and in the *Plank Position*.

The wrists get sore after doing a couple of Sun Salutations. The reason for this is often weak wrists and tight lower arm muscles. If it hurts, you should take a break, rotate the wrists, and spread out your fingers. Soreness isn't dangerous and could be a positive sign of the muscles in the lower arm being trained and strengthened. Give your lower arms massages regularly and continue training in *Sun Salutation*. Many people who suffer from arthritis in their hands and wrists get better and don't feel pain anymore thanks to yoga. People who suffer from Reynold's Syndrome (muscles often freeze around the fingers, feet, and nose—and fingertips often get white and numb when it is cold) get better from regularly doing yoga because of the increase in blood circulation.

The loin and the lower part of the back hurt. If you suffer from chronic back pains or minor back problems after an injury, training, stress, or sedentary work, it is easy to make mistakes in *Upward Facing Dog*. Avoid dropping your back (swaying) by keeping your knees on the mat and making yourself heavy in the hips. Concentrate on keeping the stomach tightened.

My feet hurt when I do Upward Facing Dog. This is often the result of a contraction in the foot muscles and in the Achilles' tendon, and there's a risk of getting "ballet feet." This is common. When the soles of the feet are pointing upwards, the top side of the foot is stretched out. Take it easy.

My knees hurt. The Dog sequence is good training for weak or injured knees because you are stretching and tightening the front and back sides of the thigh, as well as the calf muscles and the shinbone. This process helps the legs find their natural balance. Be careful about how you place your feet (parallel) and how you're standing. If you're resting more on the inner side of the foot, for instance when standing in *Tadasana*, you probably have an imbalance in your knees. Try to put the weight on the outer side (not the arch, as then you'll be knock-kneed).

Surya Namaskara B: Sun Salutation B

Sun Salutation B adds two new poses: *the Chair Pose (Utkatasana)* and *Warrior Pose A (Virabhadrasana)*. They work deep into the hip area and make posture and concentration stronger. *Sun Salutation B* increases body heat and prepares the body for the next step. *Sun Salutation* A, followed by *Sun Salutation B*, is the basis of yoga training.

Train the *Sun Salutations* until you can move continuously with ease and with the right technique between the poses. This usually takes between three and four weeks of regular training, at least four times a week. If you are a beginner, it is a good idea to do 30 minutes of *Sun Salutations* as well as relaxation exercises like *the Plough* (page 109) followed by *the Fish* (page 111) and *Corpse Pose* (page 112) as often as you can. It will make you stronger and improve your breathing techniques and concentration before you start doing the standing poses. Stick to this chapter and continue the work. When you are ready to move on, the last exhalation in *Sun Salutation B* is followed by the first movement in the standing pose *Side Plank Pose* (page 81)

If you feel pain in your back or knees after *Warrior Pose*, you are either using the wrong technique, or you are moving forward too quickly. Avoid swaying but keep the back straight, tighten the stomach, and shoot the chest outwards. Concentrate on keeping the back leg stretched.

Surya Namaskara B: Sun Salutation B

Is shown as a sequence. Each individual exercise will be explained on the following pages.

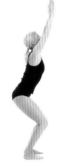
1. The Chair Pose

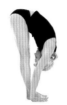
2. Head to Knee

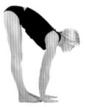
3. Look Up

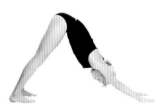
4. Downward Facing Dog

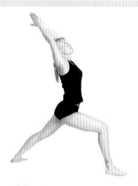
8. Warrior pose A, right leg

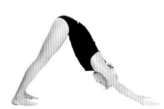
9. Downward Facing Dog

10. The Plank Position

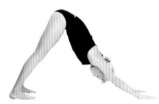
14. Downward Facing Dog

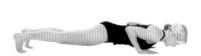
15. The Plank Position

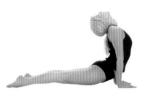
16. Upward Facing Dog

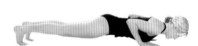

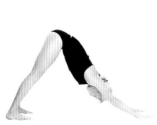

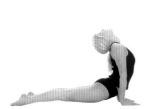

5. The Plank Position

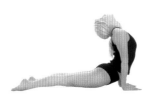

6. Upward Facing Dog

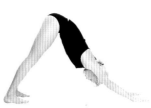

7. Downward Facing Dog

11. Upward Facing Dog

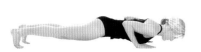

12. Downward Facing Dog

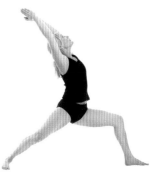

13. Warrior Pose A, left leg

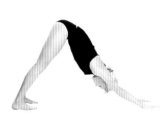

17. Downward Facing Dog

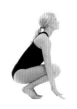

18. Squatting Pose—look up

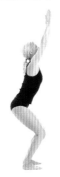

19. The Chair Pose

Utkatasana: The Chair Pose

Begins with Sama-sthiti, initiates Sun Salutaion B, and is followed by Head to Knee.

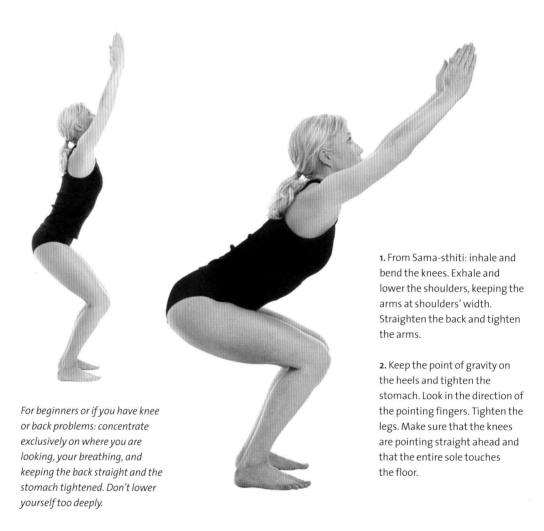

1. From Sama-sthiti: inhale and bend the knees. Exhale and lower the shoulders, keeping the arms at shoulders' width. Straighten the back and tighten the arms.

2. Keep the point of gravity on the heels and tighten the stomach. Look in the direction of the pointing fingers. Tighten the legs. Make sure that the knees are pointing straight ahead and that the entire sole touches the floor.

For beginners or if you have knee or back problems: concentrate exclusively on where you are looking, your breathing, and keeping the back straight and the stomach tightened. Don't lower yourself too deeply.

This pose strengthens the legs, stomach, arms, calf muscles, and the area around the knees. At the same time it focuses your balance and concentration. The joints of the body get stronger and revitalized. This can counteract, ease, and prevent both rheumatism and arthritis. It's believed that in this exercise the body is united with Earth's energy at the bottom of the spine. This energy rises up through the spine and increases circulation and the body's natural power.

Virabhadrasana A: Warrior Pose A

Begins with Downward Facing Dog and is followed by Downward Facing Dog.

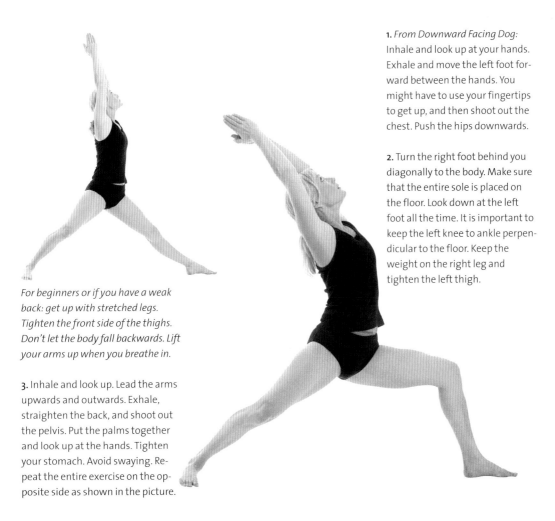

1. *From Downward Facing Dog:* Inhale and look up at your hands. Exhale and move the left foot forward between the hands. You might have to use your fingertips to get up, and then shoot out the chest. Push the hips downwards.

2. Turn the right foot behind you diagonally to the body. Make sure that the entire sole is placed on the floor. Look down at the left foot all the time. It is important to keep the left knee to ankle perpendicular to the floor. Keep the weight on the right leg and tighten the left thigh.

For beginners or if you have a weak back: get up with stretched legs. Tighten the front side of the thighs. Don't let the body fall backwards. Lift your arms up when you breathe in.

3. Inhale and look up. Lead the arms upwards and outwards. Exhale, straighten the back, and shoot out the pelvis. Put the palms together and look up at the hands. Tighten your stomach. Avoid swaying. Repeat the entire exercise on the opposite side as shown in the picture.

If you aren't leaning forward enough on your foot, you can perform a simpler version in which you place the foot as far away from you as you can. It is okay to use your hands for help. Take it easy. Don't bend in the back. Keep it tightened and straight. Keep up your breathing the entire time.

The *Warrior Poses* have a dynamic appearance, and their purpose is to increase positive attitude and give you physical control. The *Warrior Poses* are the foundation of all standing poses, and therefore it is important to master correct body posture. Keep the spine as straight as possible and shoot out the chest.

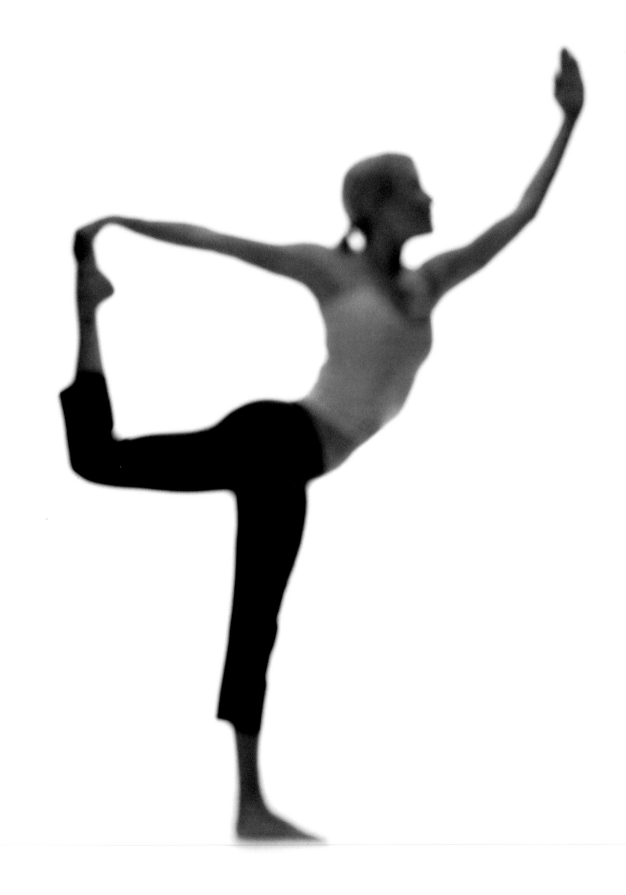

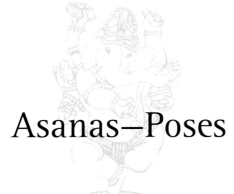

Asanas—Poses

Not until you succeed in being really flexible and soft, can you become really strong and forceful. — Zen Buddhist proverb

Standing poses

Standing poses develop strength and power. They give you a perfect posture, self-awareness, balance, presence, and involvement. When you do the standing poses, you can tell that they require your full attention in the phase between the hard and the soft parts, and between contraction (tension) and expansion (stretching out). You will find that when you lose balance, stop breathing, or lose your posture, it happens when you begin to think about something else (the future or the past). Standing poses teach us to be focused on the present. That process will, in time, make us feel how different parts of the body (including the five senses) work together to manage certain exercises and to keep our balance. If this sounds like a philosophical description of a physical activity, that's exactly what it is!

Kundalini—primordial power

If you think of the chakra system, you might ask yourself whether or not you can concentrate on the different chakras during training. You can't do so consciously. Sometimes you can do it to improve your mental training, but this only takes place on an advanced level.

If too much prana is flowing through the channels, *nadis* (page 37), it might awaken our primordial power, *Kundalini*. Kundalini is a latent universal energy in all living things. In yoga teachings, this power is symbolized in the snake that is placed at the Root Chakra, *Muladhara Chakra*. Here it blocks the door to the deepest channel in our spine, *Sushumna Nadi*. When the snake is woken up, it creeps slowly up the spine and sends cosmic energy upwards in the body. This releases tension and stress from the body and you feel incredibly strong, vital, and free. This energy can sometimes be stored throughout life, but also in different chakras for shorter periods of time. In Power Yoga the movements, poses, and breathing rouse this primordial power, helping you to be attentive towards others and yourself. If you're a beginner, you're not thinking of either streams of prana or Kundalini Power. First and foremost, you're concentrating on creating body heat in order to prevent the muscles on the back of the legs from hurting when you stretch them. You can only reach the theories beyond rote practice by performing the exercises. According to *Yoga Korunta* (page 33), asanas should never be done without a following movement: *Sloka vinya vinyasa din nakraeayet*—"Oh, yogis, don't ever do asana without vinyasa."

Vinyasa

Power Yoga is based on maintaining a flowing movement using breathing as an engine. This structure is created from different movement sequences, *Vinyasa*. Here the movement is initiated with the purpose of creating heat and concentration. *Dog in Vinyasa* (the sequence *Downward Facing Dog, the Plank Position, Upward Facing Dog* to *Downward Facing Dog*—pages 64–65, movements 6–9) is a typical example of *Vinyasa*, and it runs like a thread through the entire physical structure of Power Yoga. On the following pages (pages 81–84), *Dog in Vinyasa* will link some of the poses together.

WARNING

Do the exercises in this chapter a couple of times a week, but make sure always to start with *Sun Salutation* A and B and finish with relaxation. It is highly recommended that *the Plough, the Fish,* and *Corpse Pose* are part of the closing sequence of the training (pages 109–112). The development of these exercises can take longer for some people than others. Work slowly and with care on each asana and listen to your breathing. It is very important that you pay attention to the signals your body is sending you. These signals tell you how far you can go in each exercise.

Vasisthasana: Side Plank Pose

Begins with the Downward Facing Dog and is followed by Dog in Vinyasa.

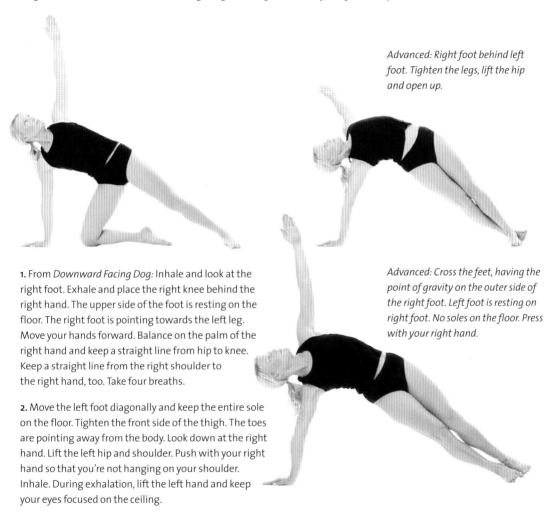

Advanced: Right foot behind left foot. Tighten the legs, lift the hip and open up.

1. From *Downward Facing Dog:* Inhale and look at the right foot. Exhale and place the right knee behind the right hand. The upper side of the foot is resting on the floor. The right foot is pointing towards the left leg. Move your hands forward. Balance on the palm of the right hand and keep a straight line from hip to knee. Keep a straight line from the right shoulder to the right hand, too. Take four breaths.

2. Move the left foot diagonally and keep the entire sole on the floor. Tighten the front side of the thigh. The toes are pointing away from the body. Look down at the right hand. Lift the left hip and shoulder. Push with your right hand so that you're not hanging on your shoulder. Inhale. During exhalation, lift the left hand and keep your eyes focused on the ceiling.

Advanced: Cross the feet, having the point of gravity on the outer side of the right foot. Left foot is resting on right foot. No soles on the floor. Press with your right hand.

Try opening the hip and the chest towards the ceiling. Look up and focus on a point. Stay up there and breathe. Focus on a point on the floor if this puts a strain on your neck. Feel how the left side and the chest are stretched. Inhale. When you exhale, slowly bring back the left arm and place it shoulders' width from your right hand. Look at your hands. Return to *Downward Facing Dog* (page 68). Do *Dog in Vinyasa* (page 80). Repeat *Side Plank Pose* (above) on the other leg.

Prasarita Uttanasana: Intense Head to Knee

Begins with Downward Facing Dog and is followed by Dog in Vinyasa and Tadasana.

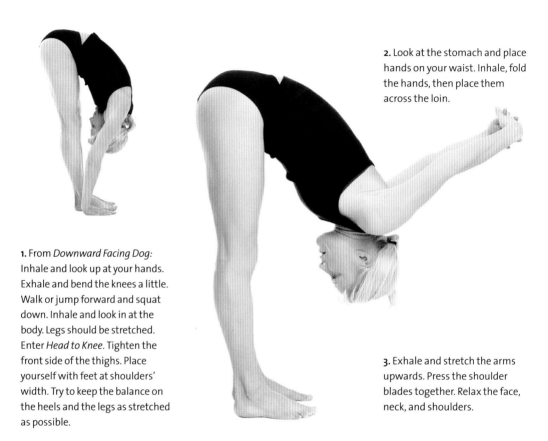

1. From *Downward Facing Dog:* Inhale and look up at your hands. Exhale and bend the knees a little. Walk or jump forward and squat down. Inhale and look in at the body. Legs should be stretched. Enter *Head to Knee*. Tighten the front side of the thighs. Place yourself with feet at shoulders' width. Try to keep the balance on the heels and the legs as stretched as possible.

2. Look at the stomach and place hands on your waist. Inhale, fold the hands, then place them across the loin.

3. Exhale and stretch the arms upwards. Press the shoulder blades together. Relax the face, neck, and shoulders.

Tighten the arms, close the eyes, and listen to your breathing. Relax the facial muscles and take a deep breath. Emit a powerful exhalation. Tension and stress in the muscles around shoulders, neck, chest, back, and face are released. The immune system gets stronger, the sinuses are cleared, and the mind and the muscles gain stamina.

Crossing to the next asanas (page 83): inhale and place hands on your waist. Slowly lower the arms to the floor. Inhale, tighten the stomach, bend the knees a little, and roll up slowly in your back. While still looking at the floor, return to *Tadasana*.

Tiriyaka Tadasana: Standing Side Bend Pose

Begins with Intense Head to Knee and is followed by Back Bend.

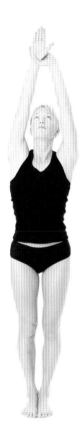

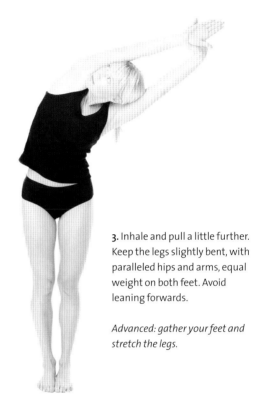

1. Inhale and stretch the arms above the head at shoulders' width, thumbs against each other. Tighten arms and hands. Exhale. Inhale and hold the wrist of the right hand with your left hand. Pull the arm towards the ears. Look at the ceiling and relax the shoulders. Exhale. Tighten the front side of the thighs.

For beginners or if you suffer from back problems: bend the knees a little and press the pelvis forward. Stand with feet at hips' width, weight placed on both feet.

2. Exhale and bend the upper body in the direction of the thumbs. Stop and look up under the arms. Inhale and carefully pull the left arm away from the body.

3. Inhale and pull a little further. Keep the legs slightly bent, with paralleled hips and arms, equal weight on both feet. Avoid leaning forwards.

Advanced: gather your feet and stretch the legs.

It is only the upper body that moves to the side in this exercise! It is important to tighten the legs and look up under the arm towards the ceiling. Keep the arms straight. Try to relax the shoulders and breathe. Take four deep breaths. Inhale and bend the knees. Focus on the ceiling and remember to tighten the stomach. Return to *Tadasana* as slowly as possible. Exhale. Change hands and place the right hand around the wrist of the left hand. Repeat this movement on the other side.

Standing Side Bend Pose develops and trains all muscles, joints, sinews, and bodily organs. Additionally, nerves, veins, and tissue are revitalized because of the increase in oxygen absorption. This pose eases sciatica, pains in the back, and other imbalances in the loin area. The body gets stronger and mobility gets better through deep stretching—especially the hip joints, waist, and torso.

Standing Back Bend

Begins with Tadasana, is followed by Head to Knee and Dog in Vinyasa.

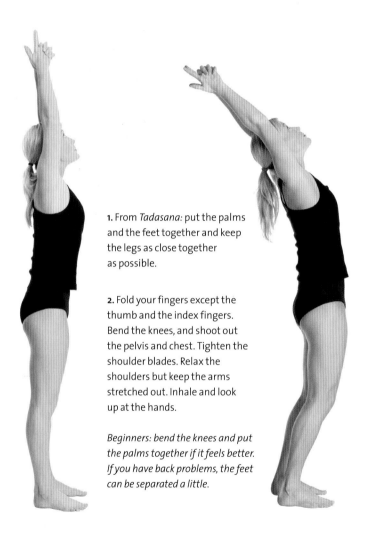

3. Exhale and let the arms fall backwards by relaxing the shoulders. Push in the opposite direction using the stomach. Concentrate on exhalation. Don't sway! If you sway, you can bend the knees a little more. Inhale and straighten up the body. Exhale and slowly enter into *Head to Knee*.

1. From *Tadasana:* put the palms and the feet together and keep the legs as close together as possible.

2. Fold your fingers except the thumb and the index fingers. Bend the knees, and shoot out the pelvis and chest. Tighten the shoulder blades. Relax the shoulders but keep the arms stretched out. Inhale and look up at the hands.

Beginners: bend the knees and put the palms together if it feels better. If you have back problems, the feet can be separated a little.

Advanced: look backwards at your fingers as far as you can. Shoot the pelvis forward; tighten the back and the stomach.

When stretching backwards, the muscles in the hip area are developed, strengthened, and stabilized. The inner organs also get stronger. This pose can ease sciatica, back pains, and other imbalances in the loin area. The strength and flexibility of the body gets better when doing deep stretching. This applies especially to the hip joints, waist, torso, and thighs.

Utthita Trikonasana: Extended Triangle Pose

Begins with Dog in Vinyasa and is followed by Triangular Twist.

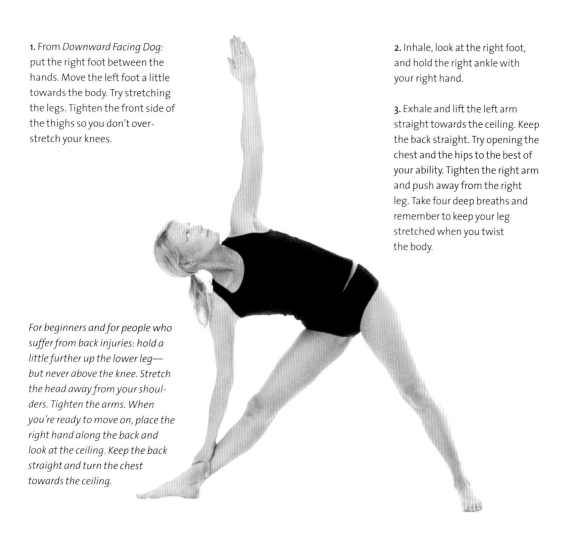

1. From *Downward Facing Dog:* put the right foot between the hands. Move the left foot a little towards the body. Try stretching the legs. Tighten the front side of the thighs so you don't over-stretch your knees.

For beginners and for people who suffer from back injuries: hold a little further up the lower leg—but never above the knee. Stretch the head away from your shoulders. Tighten the arms. When you're ready to move on, place the right hand along the back and look at the ceiling. Keep the back straight and turn the chest towards the ceiling.

2. Inhale, look at the right foot, and hold the right ankle with your right hand.

3. Exhale and lift the left arm straight towards the ceiling. Keep the back straight. Try opening the chest and the hips to the best of your ability. Tighten the right arm and push away from the right leg. Take four deep breaths and remember to keep your leg stretched when you twist the body.

Utthita means "expanding," *tri* means "three," and *kona* means "angle." *Parivritta* (page 86) means rotation. These poses can be done as standing rotation exercises. They shape the waist and legs and make them stronger, and they can ease loin problems. Rotation exercises strengthen the inner organs in the abdomen and eliminate poisonous substances.

Parivritta Trikonasana: Revolved Triangle Pose

Begins with Extended Triangle Pose and is followed by Warrior C.

1. Inhale and slowly clasp the right ankle with the left hand. Exhale and lift the right arm towards the ceiling.

2. Look at the right hand and push the left hand away. Don't forget to tighten the front side of the thighs. Remember that the hips must point towards the floor. Tighten arms, back, and stomach. Take four deep breaths. Keep looking upwards.

Beginners: try supporting with the fingertips on your shin bone if the pose is too difficult. Place the right arm along the back. Try not to bend the knees.

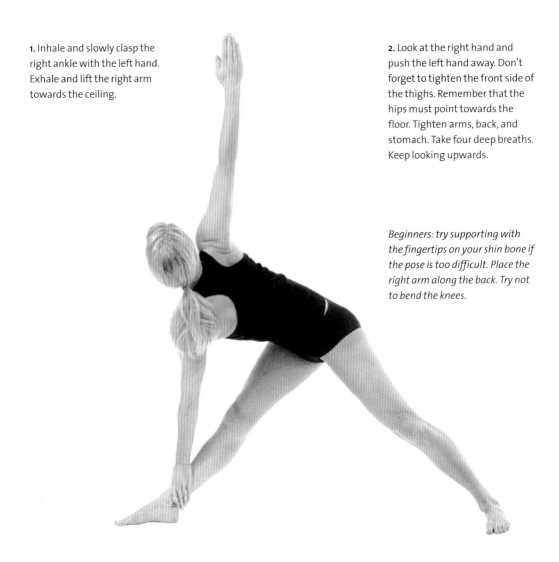

If you feel dizzy, it is a sign that waste products and poison are leaving the body. That's a good thing. The discomfort will quickly go away. If the feeling's too uncomfortable, stop the exercise and take a couple of deep breaths before trying again.

Virabhadrasana C: Warrior C

Begins with Revolved Triangle Pose and is followed by Sun Salutation A.

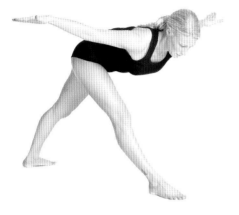

1. From *Revolved Triangle Pose:* inhale and look down at the right foot. Breathe and stretch out the arms like wings over the right leg. Palms must face the floor. Keep the back straight and tighten the muscles on the front side of the thighs. Avoid the shoulders moving towards the ears.

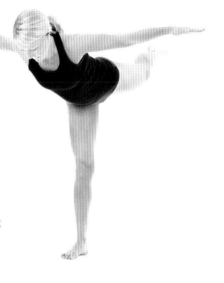

2. Exhale and focus on a point on the floor in front of you. Bend the left knee and stand on the toes on the left foot. Slowly put the body weight on the right leg. Slowly lift the left leg and tighten. Shoot the chest forward.

3. Slowly lift the left leg. Keep your eyes on the floor and breathe. Engage the shoulder blades, legs, and stomach. Lower the shoulders. Take four deep breaths focusing on exhalation.

4. If you want to move on, lead the arms slowly backwards along the sides of the body. Take two deep breaths. Exhale and turn slowly into *Tadasana.*

This pose is powerful and dynamic. Here the focus is on the mind, which helps you keep the balance on the right leg. You challenge the mind and unite your mental and physical energies. *Warrior C* gives you great strength, balance, and endurance. Congratulate yourself for each second you're able to keep standing. Breathe and concentrate all your energy on keeping the strength in the body and the breathing. A great part of the balance is focused in the upper body, in particular the chest.

Warrior C is followed by *Sun Salutation A* (pages 64–65). From *Downward Facing Dog* in Sun Salutation (exercise no. 9) repeat *Extended Triangle Pose, Revolved Triangle Pose,* and *Warrior C* (pages 85–87) on the opposite leg. Finish the sequence with *Sun Salutation* A.

Eka Pada Sirsasana: Head to Foot

Begins with Downward Facing Dog and is followed by Revolved Side Angle Pose.

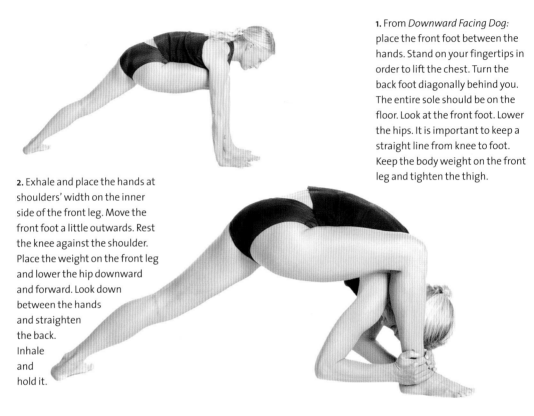

1. From *Downward Facing Dog:* place the front foot between the hands. Stand on your fingertips in order to lift the chest. Turn the back foot diagonally behind you. The entire sole should be on the floor. Look at the front foot. Lower the hips. It is important to keep a straight line from knee to foot. Keep the body weight on the front leg and tighten the thigh.

2. Exhale and place the hands at shoulders' width on the inner side of the front leg. Move the front foot a little outwards. Rest the knee against the shoulder. Place the weight on the front leg and lower the hip downward and forward. Look down between the hands and straighten the back. Inhale and hold it.

3. Exhale and calmly bend the elbows. Stop when your elbows tell you to stop. Place equal weight on both the right and left side.

It is important that the buttocks don't move backwards when you move down. It has to pull on the outer side of the hip, in the seat muscles, and on the inner side of the thighs. Pay attention to what feels right. Go all the way down on your lower arms if you can.

Eka Pada Sirsasana trains all the muscles and sinews of the body. It shapes the thighs, hips, and waist. The inner organs are stimulated and the nerves are calmed. The combination of the body's posture and the breathing balances the endocrine system (the glands) and eliminates poisonous substances from the body. If you feel dizzy, this means the poisonous substances are being eliminated from the body. Stop if you feel uncomfortable and breathe calmly to reestablish your balance.

Parivritta Parsvakonasana: Revolved Side Angle Pose

Begins with Eka Pada Sirsasana and is followed by Uttanasana.

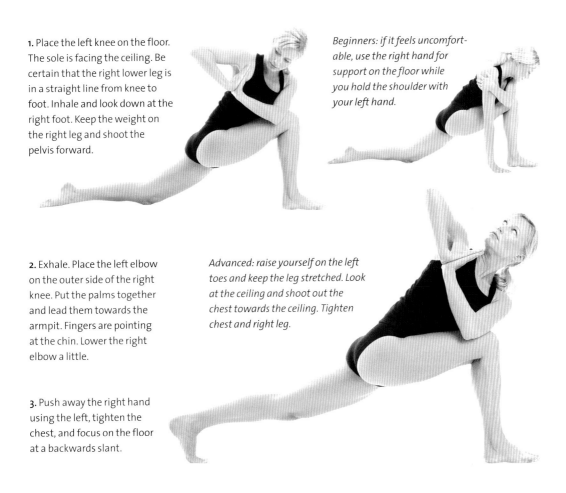

1. Place the left knee on the floor. The sole is facing the ceiling. Be certain that the right lower leg is in a straight line from knee to foot. Inhale and look down at the right foot. Keep the weight on the right leg and shoot the pelvis forward.

Beginners: if it feels uncomfortable, use the right hand for support on the floor while you hold the shoulder with your left hand.

2. Exhale. Place the left elbow on the outer side of the right knee. Put the palms together and lead them towards the armpit. Fingers are pointing at the chin. Lower the right elbow a little.

Advanced: raise yourself on the left toes and keep the leg stretched. Look at the ceiling and shoot out the chest towards the ceiling. Tighten chest and right leg.

3. Push away the right hand using the left, tighten the chest, and focus on the floor at a backwards slant.

The pose is also called "Revolved Half Tower" or the "Power Yoga Pose" because it contains all the elements of Power Yoga training: mobility, flexibility, balance, strength, and breathing. Poisonous substances are eliminated from the body in this pose. If you feel ill or dizzy, it is a sign of poisonous substances leaving the body. If you feel severe discomfort, you might have been eating or did not drink enough water just before training. You may have also had too much caffeine during the day. Take a break if you need to.

Ardha Rajakapotasana: Half Dove Pose

Begins with Revolved Side Angle Pose and is followed by Dog in Vinyasa.

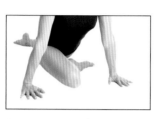

Beginners: stop and turn the heel to the left side of the groin and move your knee forwards so that the hip is pointing at the floor. Keep the back leg stretched.

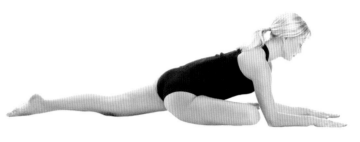

1. Inhale and place the hands on each side of the right foot. Exhale and move the hands a little and slowly turn towards the right foot using the left hand. Straighten the back and make sure that the hip is pointing at the floor so you don't slide and rest on the right side.

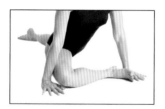

Advanced: lower the right knee and place the lower leg on the floor. Left foot is pointing towards the right hand and the left knee towards the left hand. Push the right leg a little backwards.

2. Inhale and focus on the floor in front of you. Inhale and slowly crawl forward on your hands. Stop when the body says stop. If you can, crawl forward and slowly lower the elbows to the floor. Stay in this position, close your eyes, breathe, and relax the neck. If you want to go further, you can place your forehead on the mat, stretch the arms, and relax the shoulders. Close your eyes and breathe deeply.

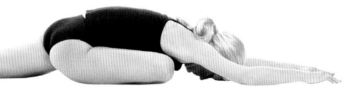

Try concentrating your breath on the area where you feel the stretch (the hips and the seat muscle). Slowly walk backwards on your hands and place them on each side of the right leg. Inhale and place the toes of the left foot on the floor. Lift the left knee from the floor, tighten chest and stomach, and focus on the floor. Exhale and push away from the floor. Return to *Downward Facing Dog* and move into *Dog in Vinyasa*. Repeat the poses *Eka Pada Sirsasana, Revolved Side Angle Pose,* and *Half Dove Pose* (page 88–90) using the opposite leg. End the sequence in *Downward Facing Dog* and *Dog in Vinyasa* (page 80).

Kundalini Virabhadrasana: Primordial Power

Begins with Half Dove Pose and Dog in Vinyasa and is followed by the Tower.

1. From *Downward Facing Dog:* inhale and look up at your hands. Exhale, walk, or jump forward and squat down. Breathe in. Look up at the ceiling and slowly rise into the standing pose with the arms hanging down the sides of the body. Roll the shoulders backwards and exhale.

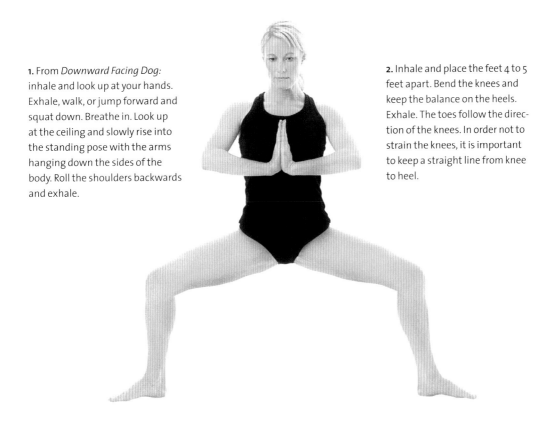

2. Inhale and place the feet 4 to 5 feet apart. Bend the knees and keep the balance on the heels. Exhale. The toes follow the direction of the knees. In order not to strain the knees, it is important to keep a straight line from knee to heel.

Tighten the stomach and keep the back straight. Lower the shoulders and shoot out the chest. Avoid swaying. Put the palms together as shown in the picture. Focus on a point on the floor. Engage all the muscles from the neck down to the toes, one area of muscles at a time. Press the hands together. Increase the power little by little. Take deep breaths and concentrate on exhalation. Be careful about your posture. Close your eyes if you can.

This pose strengthens the legs, back, stomach, and torso. Your posture and stamina improve, and *Kundalini* (page 79) is stimulated. This pose also increases mental capacity, releases inner tensions, and gives power to both body and mind.

Prasarita Padottasana: Tower A in Vinyasa

Begins with Primordial Power and is followed by Standing Bend, Downward Facing Dog, and Dog in Vinyasa.

1. From *Primordial Power:* inhale and let go of your arms. Keep the legs stretched, toes pointing forwards. Exhale and place your hands on the loin.

2. Vinyasa 1: keep the balance on the heels. Inhale, tighten the shoulder blades, and focus your eyes as far back as you can.

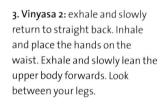

3. Vinyasa 2: exhale and slowly return to straight back. Inhale and place the hands on the waist. Exhale and slowly lean the upper body forwards. Look between your legs.

4. Vinyasa 3: Tower A. Hold the hands around the ankles. Tighten the thighs. Bend the elbows and relax the neck and shoulders. Let the head reach the floor if you can.

Beginners: hold on just below the knees. Keep your legs as stretched as possible—don't worry if you can't reach your ankles.

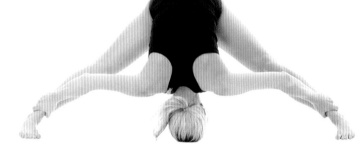

5. Inhale (still holding your ankles) and straighten your back. Relax the arms and focus on a point in front of you. Exhale and look back in again.

6. Vinyasa 4: focus on the floor and place your hands on the point you're looking at. Exhale, bend the knees and move the heels towards the body. Inhale, tighten the stomach and look in at the body. Roll up and straighten the back.

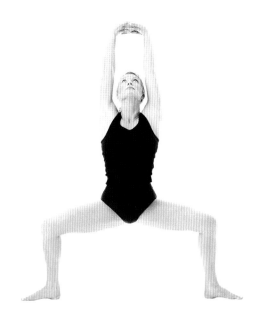

7. **Vinyasa 5:** inhale and stretch your arms towards the ceiling. Fold your hands above the head. Exhale and turn the palms towards the ceiling. The arms should make a straight line next to the ears.

8. Inhale and lower your buttocks towards the floor while you stretch the upper body upwards. Straighten the back. Imagine that the upper body is pulled upwards while the lower body is pulled downwards. Tighten the body. Take four deep breaths.

9. **Vinyasa 6:** inhale and place the elbows on the knees. Move the heels towards the body. Stand in a 90-degree angle. Keep the weight on the heels. Exhale and lower your buttocks a little more. Put the thumbs and the index fingers together. Stretch the hands away from the body.

10. **Vinyasa 7:** Inhale. Look at the ceiling. Keep the back straight. Tighten the shoulder blades and chest. Lift the head away from the shoulders. Exhale and slowly push out the legs as far as possible using your lower arms. Take four deep breaths. Tighten the legs during inhalation at the same time you're focusing on the floor in front of you. Roll up slowly to a straight back. Return to *Tadasana*.

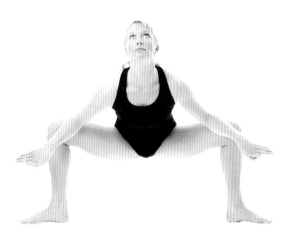

The Tower strengthens the leg muscles, builds up mobility in the spine, increases lung capacity, and allows you to breathe more deeply. It cleanses and revitalizes the inner organs in the abdomen. Stiffness in both the neck and shoulders will often completely disappear. This pose calms the central nervous system while preventing fatigue, and it increases the blood circulation.

Vrksasana: The Tree

Begins with Tadasana and is followed by Sun Salutation A.

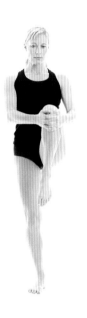

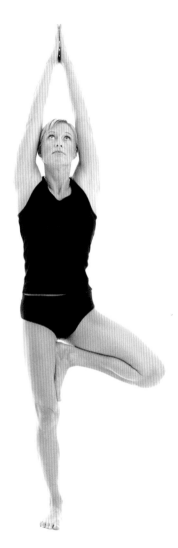

3. Tighten the right leg and shoulder blades and keep chest, arms, and stomach stretched out and tightened. Inhale and hold the left foot with the left hand. Exhale and lead the sole of the foot towards the inner side of the right thigh. Let the heel get as high up as possible and press the foot against the thigh. Keep your back straight and focus. Take four deep breaths.

Beginners: hold the left foot with the left hand and lead the right arm straight towards the ceiling. Keep the arm next to the ear.

Advanced: press the palms together in front of the chest. Stretch the arms above the head and look at the hands.

4. Hold the left foot with the left hand and pull the knee towards the chest. Push the knee towards the chest and slowly lower the leg. Repeat the same exercise on the left leg followed by *Sun Salutation A* (pages 64–65).

1. Stand with the feet at shoulders' width and keep the balance on the heels. Bend the knees a little without swaying. Tighten the stomach and straighten the back. Roll the shoulders back. Inhale and focus on a point on the floor in front of you.

2. Exhale. Place the weight on the right foot and lift the left knee towards the chest. Hold the knee with your hands.

This exercise increases positive power. It improves balance and enhances muscle stability and can help alleviate gall bladder, kidney, and pancreas problems. Just as in the other balance exercises, it is important to be very focused, *drishti,* and concentrate on breathing and posture.

Salabhasana: The Locust

Begins with Downward Facing Dog and is followed by Stomach Lift.

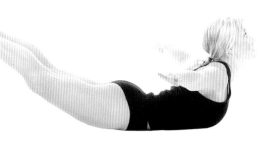

1. From *Downward Facing Dog:* inhale and look up at your hands. Exhale and lay down on your stomach. Place the feet shoulders' width apart and stretch the arms above the head at shoulders' width. Point the thumbs towards the ceiling.

2. Tighten the legs. Inhale and hold your breath. Exhale and lift arms and legs from the floor.

3. Relax in the shoulders and focus on a point at the tip of the fingers. Tighten the buttocks and the back side of the thighs. Tighten the loin. Breathe deeply. Stretch the arms out like wings.

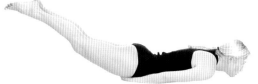

For beginners and people with back problems: lift your buttocks, place the palms against the groin and press the hips down. Let the hips rest on the hands. Relax the upper body with the chin on the floor. Inhale and lift the thighs from the floor. Keep the balance on the hips and exhale.

4. Take two breaths. Lift the chest a little from the floor if you can. Lead the arms backwards. Close your eyes and lift as high as you can. Exhale and rest the chin on the floor and place the arms down next to the body. Close your eyes and breathe.

To achieve the best result, make sure your body posture is as correct as possible. Try to avoid tenseness in your neck.

This exercise shapes the muscles in the back, seat, stomach, and arms and makes them stronger. It increases the blood circulation and raises the energy level in the body.

Pinca Mayurasana: Stomach Lift

Begins with the Locust and is followed by the Bow.

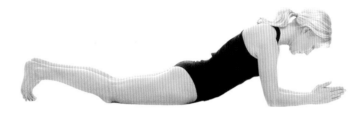

1. From the *Locust:* inhale and place yourself on your elbows. Put your toes on the floor and keep the legs close together.

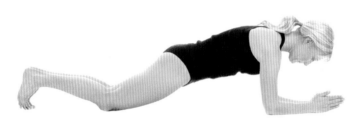

2. Exhale. Look inwards at the chest and lift the stomach from the floor. Keep shoulders and elbows in a straight line. Push the head away from the shoulders. Balance on the elbows, knees, and toes. Tighten stomach and chest. Breathe strongly with an emphasis on exhalation. Raise yourself to the knees if possible. Keep the body parallel with the floor. Hips should be heavy.

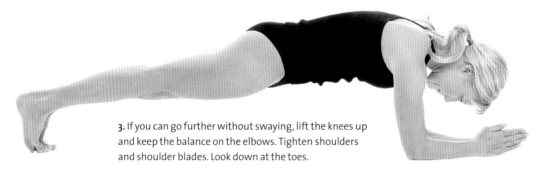

3. If you can go further without swaying, lift the knees up and keep the balance on the elbows. Tighten shoulders and shoulder blades. Look down at the toes.

When you have lifted yourself up in *Stomach Lift*, take eight deep breaths. After this, lower your knees, hips, and chest to the floor. Place yourself on the stomach with your chin on the floor and your arms next to your body.

This exercise strengthens stomach muscles, shoulders, arms, chest, and neck.

Dhanurasana: The Bow

Begins with Stomach Lift and is followed by the Camel.

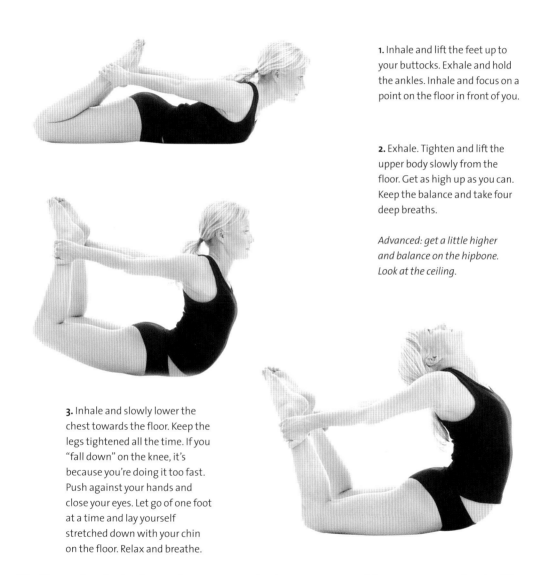

1. Inhale and lift the feet up to your buttocks. Exhale and hold the ankles. Inhale and focus on a point on the floor in front of you.

2. Exhale. Tighten and lift the upper body slowly from the floor. Get as high up as you can. Keep the balance and take four deep breaths.

Advanced: get a little higher and balance on the hipbone. Look at the ceiling.

3. Inhale and slowly lower the chest towards the floor. Keep the legs tightened all the time. If you "fall down" on the knee, it's because you're doing it too fast. Push against your hands and close your eyes. Let go of one foot at a time and lay yourself stretched down with your chin on the floor. Relax and breathe.

The Bow trains the back muscles, massages the inner organs, and increases energy levels. The stomach's position in this exercise eases digestive and intestine problems and reduces fat accumulation on the stomach and the back.

Ushtrasana: The Camel

Begins with the Bow and is followed by the Child.

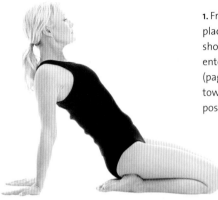

1. From *The Bow:* inhale and place the hands on the floor at shoulders' width. Exhale and enter into *Downward Facing Dog* (page 68). Lower your buttocks towards your heels. Enter seated pose and keep the back straight.

2. Pull the buttocks in so you sit on your heels. Roll the shoulders backwards and keep the legs gathered. Inhale and place the hands on the floor behind the body. The fingers must point away from the body.

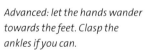

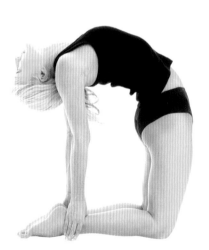

Advanced: let the hands wander towards the feet. Clasp the ankles if you can.

3. Exhale. Look up and lift the pelvis towards the ceiling. Tighten the legs. Stay here as long as possible and let the head fall back. Relax the neck and close your eyes. Take four deep breaths.

If you feel pain, you must stop the exercise and rest in *the Child* (page 99). Separate the legs if your back hurts. At the end of the exercise, inhale, move the hands back, lower the pelvis, and look at your stomach. Be careful! When the buttocks are above the heels, you slowly sit up and lead the arms in front of you to enter *the Child*.

The Bow and *the Camel* are rejuvenating. They release tension in the neck and shoulders while alleviating imbalances in your back.

Balasana: The Child

Begins with the Camel and is followed by the Boat.

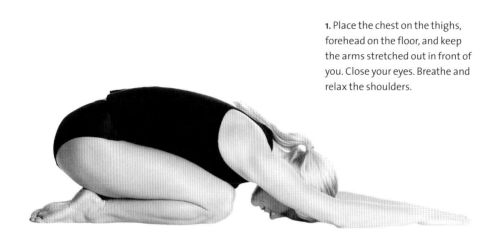

1. Place the chest on the thighs, forehead on the floor, and keep the arms stretched out in front of you. Close your eyes. Breathe and relax the shoulders.

The Child calms the nervous system and balances energy in the back, neck, and shoulders. The exercise also eases tension in the shoulder and neck area.

Seated poses

Standing pose-sequences should always be followed by a sequence of seated poses. This creates energy and strength and prepares body, soul, and mind for relaxation. Seated poses are incredibly important because they cause a natural and healthy afflux of blood to flow to the muscles and organs. Lungs, liver, heart, bowels, gall bladder and kidneys, and the autonomic nervous system are cleansed and get stronger in seated poses. Because the seated poses primarily work with strength and rotation of the upper body, calming neural signals are sent to the brain. Many of the seated asanas allow the five senses to rest while focusing and training the mind and strengthening the soul.

Paripurna Navasana: The Boat

Begins with the Camel and is followed by Full Forward Bend Pose.

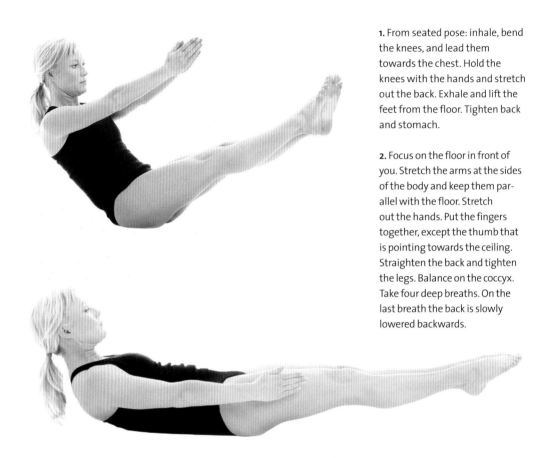

1. From seated pose: inhale, bend the knees, and lead them towards the chest. Hold the knees with the hands and stretch out the back. Exhale and lift the feet from the floor. Tighten back and stomach.

2. Focus on the floor in front of you. Stretch the arms at the sides of the body and keep them parallel with the floor. Stretch out the hands. Put the fingers together, except the thumb that is pointing towards the ceiling. Straighten the back and tighten the legs. Balance on the coccyx. Take four deep breaths. On the last breath the back is slowly lowered backwards.

3. Exhale. Keep the neck and back stretched. Tighten the stomach, bring the chest forward, and slowly lower the backside of the body towards the floor.

4. Let the body be as parallel to the floor as possible without lying down. Take two deep breaths. Return to initial pose by pulling the body together. Hold the knees without the feet touching the floor. Repeat the exercise. When you finish, put the feet on the floor.

This exercise is good for physical body balance, and it builds up strength in the back, legs, and stomach. *Navasana* also nurtures the liver and kidneys.

Paschimottanasana: Full Forward Bend Pose

Begins with the Boat and is followed by Wide-angled Seated Fold.

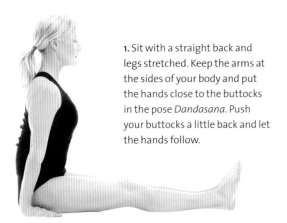

1. Sit with a straight back and legs stretched. Keep the arms at the sides of your body and put the hands close to the buttocks in the pose *Dandasana*. Push your buttocks a little back and let the hands follow.

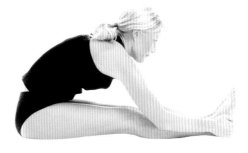

2. Inhale and place the hands on the lower legs. Exhale and clasp the ankles. Inhale and straighten the back. Focus on a point right in front of you and bend the elbows a little.

3. Inhale and bend over the legs, keeping the back as straight as possible. Imagine that the stomach is resting on the upper side of the thighs. Keep the pose and take 6–8 breaths.

Beginners: bend the knees a little if it feels better. Inhale and look at the knees. Continue like this until you reach your limit. Stay there and take six deep breaths. Slowly get back to straight back.

Advanced: clasp the feet or hold the big toes with the thumb and index finger.

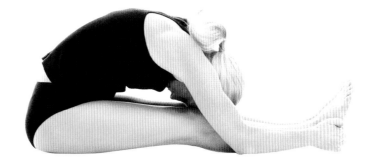

This exercise strengthens the legs and stomach muscles and increases mobility on the back sides of the thighs and in the spine. The abdominal organs are cleansed and strengthened. This asana focuses on the waistline and prevents constipation. The back is stretched intensely. The movement forward stimulates the kidneys, liver, and the pancreas because you activate stomach pressure and breathe with your diaphragm. *Paschimottanasana* can also prevent and ease depression.

Ardha Matsyendrasana: Half Lord of the Fish Pose

Begins with Full Forward Bend Pose and is followed by Half Lord of the Fish Pose.

1. Inhale and put the right foot across the left leg next to the buttocks.

2. Put the left elbow against the right knee. The fingers point away from the body. Keep your back straight and pull the knee towards your chest. Avoid letting all the body weight rest on the arm.

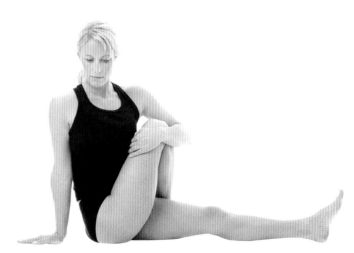

3. Raise the left hand and let the fingers point towards the ceiling. Take four deep breaths. Repeat the exercise to the left side.

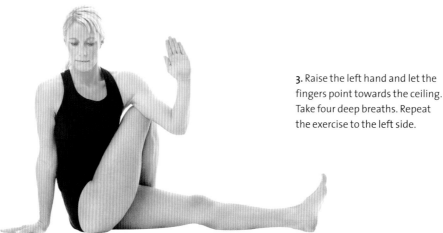

Half Lord of the Fish Pose injects a healthy afflux of blood to the abdominal organs as well as the spine. This and the following exercises are good if you suffer from back problems, tense loin muscles, liver problems, incontinence, intestine problems, pancreas problems, and constipation.

Marichyasana B: The Sage Twist

Begins with the Half Lord of the Fish Pose and is followed by Wide-angled Seated Fold.

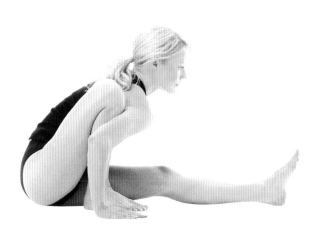

1. Inhale and put the right heel towards the buttocks. Push yourself forwards over the left thigh and exhale.

2. Inhale and place the hands on the floor on each side of the body. Let the right knee rest on the shoulder and the back side of the arm. Stay here if you're a beginner. After this, slowly return and repeat the same exercise with the left leg. Finish the exercise in *Dandasana* (page 101, step 1).

Advanced: lead the right arm backwards and around the right leg and place the left arm on the back. Put the right hand around the left wrist and put the left thumb and index finger together. Keep the other fingers straight and tightened. Take four deep breaths. After this return slowly and repeat the same exercise with the left leg. Finish in Dandasana.

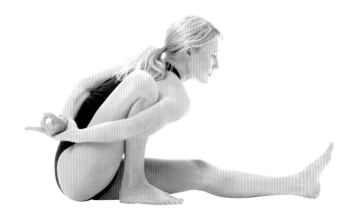

This is an advanced pose. If the exercise is too hard, move on to the next exercise. The twists you do in yoga quickly help the body alleviate loin and digestive problems. In this exercise, neck muscles are strengthened, tension and stress in the spine are eased, hip and legs get massaged, and the intestines are stimulated, aiding digestion. Additionally, the liver and spleen are energized during the exercise and the stomach gets firmer.

Upavishta Konasana: Wide-angled Seated Fold

Begins with Half Lord of the Fish Pose and is followed by Bound Angle Pose.

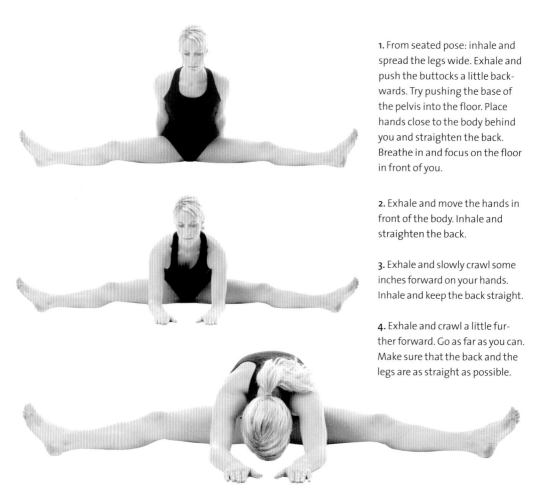

1. From seated pose: inhale and spread the legs wide. Exhale and push the buttocks a little backwards. Try pushing the base of the pelvis into the floor. Place hands close to the body behind you and straighten the back. Breathe in and focus on the floor in front of you.

2. Exhale and move the hands in front of the body. Inhale and straighten the back.

3. Exhale and slowly crawl some inches forward on your hands. Inhale and keep the back straight.

4. Exhale and crawl a little further forward. Go as far as you can. Make sure that the back and the legs are as straight as possible.

It isn't important how far down you get in this pose. When you have reached your limit, stay there and take a couple of deep breaths. Close your eyes.

Upavishta Konasna shapes the abdominal muscles and legs and makes them stronger. It also eases tension and stress in the shoulders and the chest. The thighs' back sides and the muscles around the spine get a deep stretch, and the skin gets more elastic. The exercise prevents cellulite around the buttocks and thighs.

Baddha Konasana: Bound Angle Pose

Begins with Wide-angled Seated Fold and is followed by Lateral Back Twist.

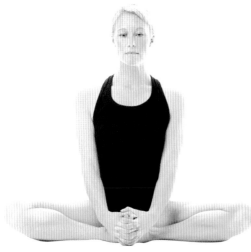

1. From seated pose: inhale. Lead the soles of the feet towards each other and pull the heels towards the base of the pelvis. Clasp the feet, straighten the back and try pushing the knees into the floor.

2. Shoot out the chest. Inhale and focus on the floor right in front of you. Fold the upper body over the legs as far down as you can. Think about pressing the stomach towards the legs using your breathing for help. Keep the back straight, tighten stomach and chest.

Advanced: if you can get the upper body all the way down without the back bending too much or the legs moving towards the ears, you can place the forehead on the floor and take eight deep breaths.

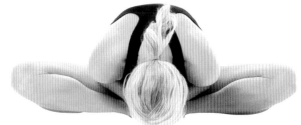

If you have problems getting the knees down to the floor, it is because you are tightening the adductors, the inward leading muscles of your inner thighs. First and foremost, work on getting the knees down and try keeping a straight back. If you can't get the upper body all the way down over the legs, that's okay. Don't start bending in the back, tightening the shoulders, or try to "look" flexible. Nobody is looking at you! It is also important to keep the weight on the buttocks—not on the knees.

The increased afflux of blood in *Baddha Konasana* cleanses the pelvic region, the lower parts of the stomach and back, and gives new energy to the kidneys, bladder, and gall bladder. It regulates the menstrual cycles and prevents and eases varicose veins, constipation, and digestive problems. This pose increases mobility in the hips, knees and thighs, and along the spine.

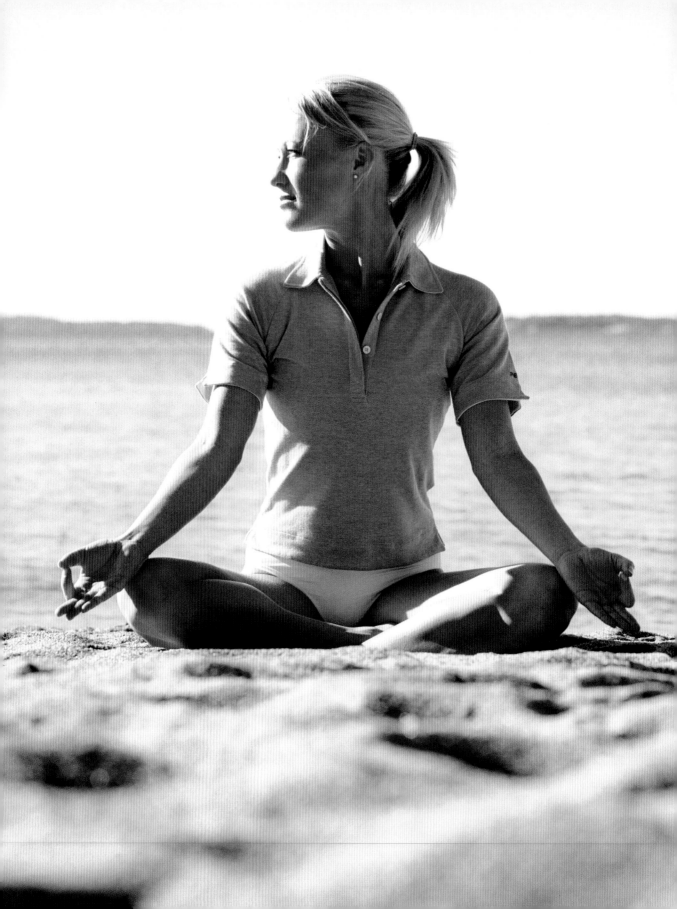

Relaxation and Meditation

There is an inner center in us where the absolute truth dwells. — Robert Browning

Relaxation sequences are incredibly important in yoga training because they give the muscles, joints, neural system, and mind the opportunity to relax, build up resistance, and recharge energy. They influence metabolism and balance the bodily system.

Note that the poses *the Plough*, *Ears Pressure Pose*, and *Shoulder Stand* should not be practiced by:

- Pregnant women. Talk to a professional yoga teacher if you have doubts or if you want advice and help to find alternative exercises. Also, some women might feel discomfort doing these exercises during their period. Avoid these exercises if that's the case. You can tell what's best for you.
- People with high blood pressure, cholesterol problems, and people who suffer from obesity.
- People who just had surgery should consult their doctor.
- People with blocks in the upper and lower part of the spine. Consult a professional yoga teacher if you feel uncertain.

Supta Pandhakonasana: Lateral Back Twist

Begins with Bound Angle Pose and is followed by the Plough and Ears Pressure Pose.

1. Lie on your back with your knees against the chest. Clasp the knees. Push the loin down and lay down the right leg.

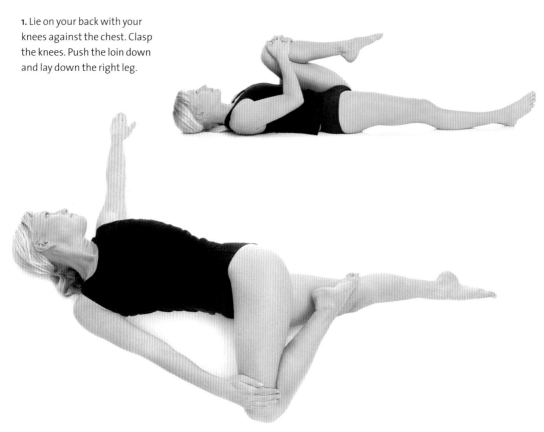

2. Inhale and put the left arm straight out to the side. Exhale and place the right hand on the outer side of the left knee. Place the left foot on the inner side of the right leg.

3. Inhale and look at the left hand. Exhale and slowly push the left knee towards the floor as far as you can, but keep the shoulders on the floor. Take four deep breaths. Repeat the exercise to the other side.

Try to close your eyes and concentrate on breathing. Concentrate on moving the mental focus to the loin.

This pose eases tensions and muscular stress in neck and shoulders, along the spine, and in the loin.

Halasana: The Plough

Begins with Lateral Back Twist and is followed by Shoulder Stand.

1. Lie on the back with the knees against the chest. Put the arms down next to the body with the palms facing the floor. Breathe in and lift the feet towards the ceiling.

2. Exhale and use the hands to push away so that the legs roll up over you. Try to get the toes to touch the floor. You can add support with the hands on the back.

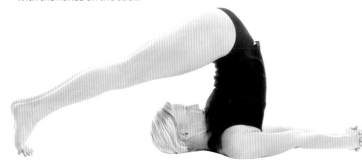

3. If you can continue from here, try to "walk" with the shoulders until you get up on your neck. Look at the chest. Take five deep breaths.

Advanced: stretch the legs and fold the hands behind the back and place the arms on the mat.

The Plough stretches the entire body, and it increases mobility in the spine to the fullest. It strengthens both the legs and the abdominal muscles. This pose stimulates and balances the activity in the thyroid gland, stabilizing your weight and regulating the menstrual cycle.

Karnapidasana: Ears Pressure Pose

Begins with the Plough and is followed by Shoulderstand.

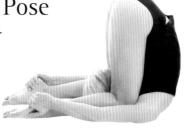

Beginners should avoid this exercise.
Inhale and bend the knees. Exhale and put the knees next to the ears. Clasp the feet. Take five deep breaths.

Salamba Sarvangasana: Shoulder Stand

Begins with the Plough or Ears Pressure Pose and is followed by the Fish.

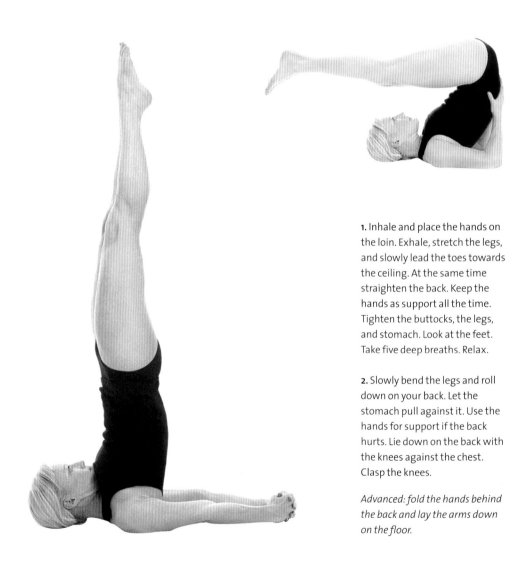

1. Inhale and place the hands on the loin. Exhale, stretch the legs, and slowly lead the toes towards the ceiling. At the same time straighten the back. Keep the hands as support all the time. Tighten the buttocks, the legs, and stomach. Look at the feet. Take five deep breaths. Relax.

2. Slowly bend the legs and roll down on your back. Let the stomach pull against it. Use the hands for support if the back hurts. Lie down on the back with the knees against the chest. Clasp the knees.

Advanced: fold the hands behind the back and lay the arms down on the floor.

This pose is one of the most important in classical yoga. It stimulates the body glands and cleans the intestines of waste products.

Matsyasana: The Fish

Begins with Shoulder Stand and is followed by Corpse Pose.

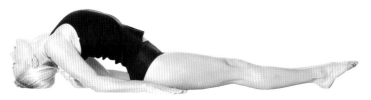

1. Inhale and lower one leg at a time. Keep the arms close to the body. Push the elbows into the floor. Exhale.

2. Inhale. Lift the chest and look backwards. Get the head all the way up. Exhale and tighten the stomach. Close the eyes if you want to.

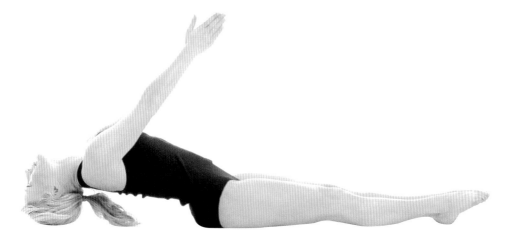

3. You can support yourself with the elbows. Take five deep breaths and slide slowly backwards. Don't try to roll but hold back using the elbows.

Advanced: put the palms together in front of the body and stretch the arms.

This exercise is just like *Shoulder Stand* and *the Plough* in that it's necessary to perform if you want to achieve maximum balance in the body. It strengthens and shapes the stomach and leg muscles, alleviates tension and stress in the neck and shoulders, increases blood circulation to the face, and increases your lung capacity when the chest is opened.

Savasana: Corpse Pose

Begins with the Fish and is followed by the Lotus Pose.

1. Lower the legs one at a time and lie down stretched out with the arms next to the body. Press down the loin towards the floor. Gather the shoulder blades and lift the chin towards the ceiling.

2. Gather the heels and let the feet fall out to the sides. Turn the hands so the palms face the ceiling. Take a deep breath and close the eyes.

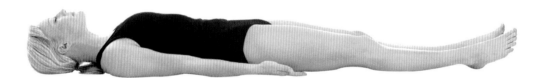

Now you can reward yourself with minutes of wonderful rest. Your body has been working hard. Keep on breathing calmly as you relax each muscle — in your face, hands, and feet. When you relax in *Corpse Pose*, the mind is allowed to rest. Think of Newton's third law: *for every action, there is an equal and opposite reaction.* Try focusing on the diaphragm. Each time you exhale, the muscles let go of stress and tension piece by piece. After this, focus on your feet. Tighten the muscles when you inhale and relax when you exhale. Do the same with the hands, and feel how you relax more and more of your body. Try to relax your face and take deep breaths. Concentrate on mental images like a beautiful deserted beach, a jungle, mountaintops, or a peaceful ocean. Lay like this for several minutes (preferably fifteen).

Inhale and lift one knee at a time towards the chest. Keep your eyes closed. Exhale and push the knees down on the chest at the same time as you're pushing the loin down. Inhale. Exhale and slowly enter *the Lotus Pose* with your eyes closed if you can. Straighten the back and push the shoulders back. Shoot out the chest. Keep your hands on the knees. Put thumb and index finger together and turn the palms towards the ceiling. Take a deep breath. Put the palms together in front of the chest/heart and relax the arms. Look down at the hands and say *Namaste*[23].

Your well-being depends on your ability to relax. The techniques you have used rejuvenate the body, reduce stress and tension in the muscles, and they calm down the nervous system. If you use the breathing techniques you have learned in your everyday life, they will refresh both body and soul. If you use them before bedtime, you will find it easier to fall and stay asleep.

In yoga asanas, the poses work like oil in the body. They make muscles and joints move easily and flexibly, strengthen all the inner organs and increase circulation without causing tiredness. The body is calmed down in complete relaxation while Pranayama, or the yoga breathing, increases prana, the electric stream—life energy. You get fuel from food, water and the air that you breathe. Finally you can make use of meditation that calms the mind, the chauffeur of the body.—Swami Vishnu Devananda

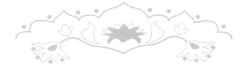

Meditation

Meditation is a central part of yoga. It makes the mind focus in a way that allows the body to rest at the same time as it's working. Meditation calls for silent reflection and is often described as an interruption of the common mental activity, or as a way of turning the Theta waves in the mind into Alfa-waves. The amplitude of the Alfa-waves is lower. When you find yourself in a meditative state, the brain waves are lowered. Meditation resembles sleep when it comes to frequency and amplitude (brain waves).

Why meditation? There are a lot of reasons, all valid. • You get in touch with reality. • It is an opportunity for unconscious reflection. • You get in touch with your inner self. • The so-called brain roar disappears, and you can hear yourself think. • It is calming and feels good. The mind and the body are resting together, and that makes you feel better. • It reduces stress and the chemical processes that make you angry and bitter. • Gives time for healing. • Positive images and thoughts come to life.

You can't force meditation. It is spontaneous. Likewise, you can't learn how to meditate, but you can learn meditation techniques. There are many different types of meditation. In northern Southeast Asia, it is common to listen to sounds from nature. For instance, if you hear a bird, you can concentrate on the sounds of birds singing and adapt the bird's energy in each breath. You are letting yourself be filled with a sense of participation and appreciation of life in the moment. In Zen Buddhism you count your breathing rhythms until you find yourself in a meditative state. This is a very popular technique, and many practice it.

Another popular technique in yoga, especially in India, is to repeat a mantra. The word *man* means "to think, fantasise, believe," and a mantra is a thought or a feeling expressed in a word. It can be a single word or a combination of sounds. The *OM*-sound is the oldest and most frequently used yoga mantra. This syllable symbolizes the universal power both in Buddhist and Hindu tradition. When you meditate, you are usually sitting in *Padmasana*—the Lotus Pose—with the hands on the knees, thumb and index finger put together, and the palms pointing towards the ceiling. If you have decided to try the mantra technique, you mustn't be afraid of your own voice! It might seem a little strange, but try to feel what happens to your body and mind. Treat it as training for your diaphragm! Start splitting the word into parts. First hum an "ah" sound, then an "oo" sound and finally an "mm" sound. End up in a nasal humming. Train each sound individually at first. After that, take a deep breath through the nose with your mouth closed. Then say "oo," exhale and say "mm". Use the diaphragm (and bandhas, if you're trained). After this, try saying "om" when you exhale. Close the eyes and continue. Every time thoughts intrude—and that will probably happen many times in the beginning—you must try to concentrate on the sound and the breathing. Let it take some time, and don't anticipate that you can meditate the first time you try it. You probably won't succeed even after trying a number of times. When it comes to how much time you should set aside, there's no time limit, but start by setting a timer to 30 to 40 minutes. Some people meditate for two minutes and others for a half or a whole hour. It's always a good idea, though, to do some meditation just after doing yoga—in the morning or in the middle of the day.

The universe and the thought are made of the same matter—they can both create confusion, and they possess enormous powers that aren't tangible.—Sir Arthur Eddington

[23] *Namaste is the name on the hand pose in itself: palm to palm. In Sanskrit it means: "I bow to the divine in you." It refers to the true self. In yoga training, you can say that you humbly give thanks to the work you have just been doing with yourself.*

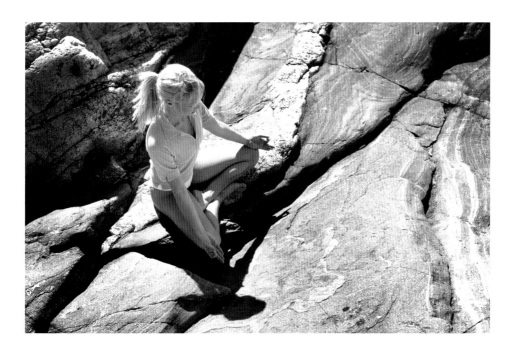

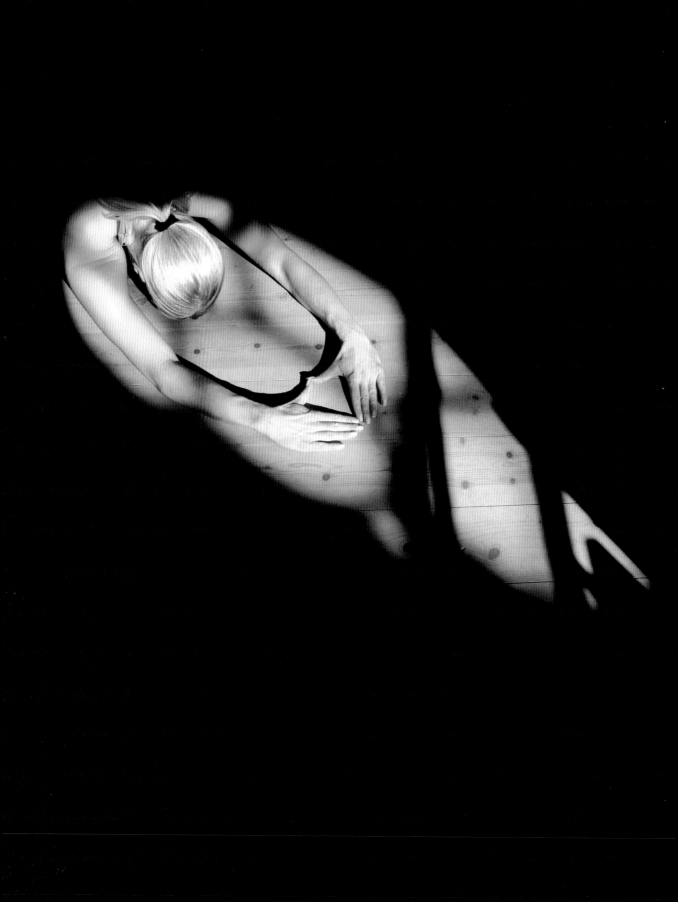

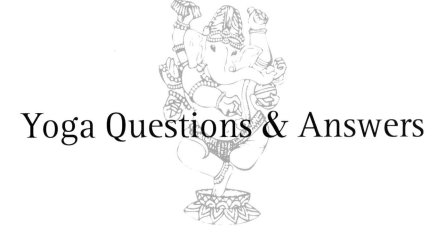

Yoga Questions & Answers

You are what you think. — Buddha

Why yoga? People all over the world practice yoga for many different kinds of reasons. Some do it to become fit, lose weight, keep in shape, balance their nervous system, calm a stressful mind, learn how to unwind, or to increase physical endurance and strength. Others perform yoga to achieve a higher sense of self, to seek answers to spiritual questions, improve their immune system, cleanse their body, and to live a more meaningful life. The goals are individual, and the yoga type you choose depends on what kind of person you are.

Thousands of years ago the wise yoga masters discovered that we couldn't unite with life before we find a source to happiness beyond desires and pain. This means that even though a person is healthy, has a balanced nervous system, and lives a meaningful life, he or she can nevertheless feel that happiness isn't present. You have to penetrate through several layers that limit you before you can achieve true happiness in your heart, body, and mind.

The highest goal is to become one with yourself and all living things, as well as to cleanse your heart, mind, and body of the impurities that disturb individual growth. Regardless of what the reason might be for you doing yoga, it is good to know something about the philosophy of yoga. This knowledge gives you the opportunity to complete your journey towards being a completely fulfilled human being. Yoga accommodates the facts that we're all different individuals, value different things, and have different shapes by offering movements and paces that are specifically right for each of us.

What is a guru? The word comes from Sanskrit. In Sanskrit, *guru* means "meaningful" and "big." A guru is a great teacher, someone whose advice is important for us to learn. The syllable *gu* represents darkness and the syllable *ru* "remove." A guru removes the spiritual darkness. If you're primarily interested in learning poses, movements, and breathing techniques, it is enough to have a qualified yoga teacher. On the other hand, if you've chosen yoga as a spiritual path, it might be a good idea to get help from a guru. You can't find a guru in the phone book. Yoga tradition claims that *the guru finds you when the time is ripe and when you are ripe.*

Is there any age limit if you want to practice yoga? No! Anyone, no matter how old they are, can do yoga. Most mothers and fathers who do yoga at home soon find that their kids are curious, imitate the exercises, and have a great time when they actually perform *the Dog, the Crocodile,* or *the Camel* with mom and dad. It is, however, important that they meet yoga out of free will and curiosity, not because they are forced to. Children of different ages can experience great joy from practicing yoga. In my yoga groups, people from 16 to 84 participate—people of different skin colors, genders, sexual preferences, social and work statuses, as well as religious and political convictions.

How did the yoga poses and the movements get their names? Unfortunately there are no specific originators for these names, but the poses have been developed in different periods throughout yoga's history. Yoga is an oral tradition, and insight and wisdom have been passed down from master to student over thousands of years. The names have different connections to the poses. Some names describe the shape that the body looks like during the exercise, like the *Triangle Pose*. The name might also point to the way the body works, like *Head to Knee*. Many of the names have been taken from nature (for instance, the *Mountain Pose*, as well as *the Dog, the Camel* and *the Turtle*) or from celestial bodies like *the Sun* and *the Moon*. Other names stem from comparing the pose with objects—for instance *the Plough*, *the Bow*, and *the Bridge*. Some exercises are named after masters, such as the *Bharadvaja* and *Goraksa*. Furthermore, there is the part of the name that reminds us why we are actually performing a movement: freedom, skill, and pleasure. There are also some names that contain different phases of our own lives, like the *Embryo*, *Corpse Pose*, *the Child*, and so forth. Even though the names are part of a tradition, they might vary in their execution in different yoga manuals.

How many poses are there and how many should I learn? In one of the classical yoga manuals, *Gheranda Samhita*, Geranda mentions that there are 840,000 movements—one for each single creature. He believes that only 84 movements are accessible to people and mentions 32 of them as physically useful. In modern yoga books and manuals, the number of useful poses varies, but usually there are between 30 and 40. B.K.S. Iyengar's book *Light on Yoga* describes 200, but more than half of them are very advanced, and the writer himself didn't master them until he had trained for many years. Beginners normally learn 25 to 30 poses, and that is more than enough. A yoga teacher is the best way to learn how to do yoga poses correctly, but there are many helpful books and training videos on the market as well.

Which texts are essential if I want to study classical yoga literature?
- *Yoga Sutras* by Patanjali. It has been translated into many languages and most of them have good commentaries.
- *Hathayoga Pradipika* by Yogendra. A classical Hatha Yoga manual that gives you insight into the philosophy behind physical yoga.
- *Bhagavad-Gita*. The Hindu "bible." There are many English translations of this book available.

How important is yoga theory? Very. Yoga is an interaction between theory and praxis. To achieve your maximum potential, you must study the theory. This helps you gain insight and knowledge and leads to true happiness.

Can I perform yoga if I have physical problems or have a cold? Basically, anybody can do yoga. People who have a handicap or other physical limitations can gain a lot from yoga, but they need to choose a type that is gentler, or consult a yoga teacher who can adjust the movements and the meditation techniques so they fit that individual. Many yoga schools all over the world offer special courses in yoga for either physically and mentally handicapped students. There are courses for the blind, deaf, and people who suffer from back injuries. If you suffer from an injury, limited mobility, or depression, and you feel insecure about whether or not it would be good for you to practice yoga or Power Yoga, you should talk to a yoga teacher *before* participating. Explain how you feel and listen to what the teacher says.

It is not dangerous to practice yoga if you have a cold, but you should avoid training if you're running a fever or feel really ill. The body needs rest. If you have doubts, consult a yoga teacher or your doctor. If you feel that there are exercises you can't do, then don't — or ask for an alternative. Remember that all progress takes time.

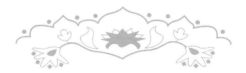

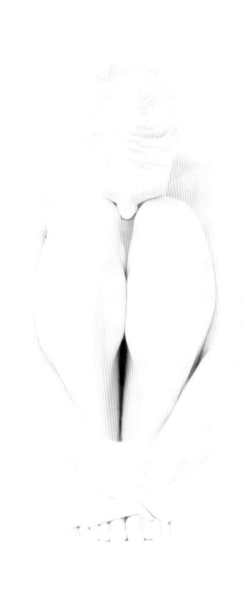

Postscript

Yoga is a fantastic system that—if you train seriously—can lead to a healthier and happier life. To me, yoga is an essential part of everyday life, a bond that grows stronger in me since I was introduced to it in 1994. It helps me in my job, when doing other kinds of physical training, and has turned me into a vital person. When I look back on my development, I can tell that yoga, as well as the study of Zen Buddhism, has taught me to be aware of the small things in life, to appreciate each and every moment. I'm more present in the moment than I used to be. Yoga training over many years has also caused better results during other kinds of training. It has given me more stamina and increased my mobility and flexibility. I haven't made drastic changes in my life, but have instead learned how to adjust and control my power in order to reach a more harmonious balance in life. Today, I work *with* my body, soul, and thoughts instead of working against them like I used to. I have found inner peace and gained a strong intuition through reflection, relaxation, and meditation. I have achieved a strong self-confidence after handling the physical and psychological hurdles that yoga has challenged me with.

As a result of working with a lot of people in my classes, I believe it is important to adjust the poses so they fit the individual, not the other way around. This is especially important in the beginning. My experience as a teacher has shown me that if you try to fit the individual to the various poses, misinterpretations happen and injuries occur more frequently. We can't blame the poses for that. This is our own fault. We sometimes tend to push ourselves too hard when we exercise and don't always pay attention to the signals that our body, mind, and soul send us. We need to learn how to listen before we can act in a careful way. Asanas and focusing on our breath can help us in this. It is also important to take one step at a time. I believe there is a lot to gain from gradually learning a pose instead of rushing through too many sequences. Rushing will only wear you out.

When I was asked to write this book, a lot of thoughts and emotions went through me before I agreed. I have so much respect for the yoga tradition, and there are many teachers out there who have so much more experience in this field than I do, but the ray of light landed on me for a reason, probably because I work both as a writer and a yoga teacher. It has been my ambition to find a balance between being true to the yoga system and trying to write a friendly and accessible book on yoga and Power Yoga. Looking back, it has been an honor to try and describe this wonderful type of yoga that today positively changes and evolves human beings to such a great extent. I hope you as a reader have found this book inspiring and that after reading it you feel motivated to start your own yoga quest.

I wish to thank some of the fantastic people that surround me. First and foremost I want to thank you, Magnus, my life friend, for the enormous love and support you show me. I wouldn't be the person I am or do what I do without my wonderful parents, my sisters, and my amazing grandmother. THANKS for being there and for all your support!

Furthermore, I want to express my gratitude towards the following people: Andreas Lundberg and Alexandra Frank for your enormous creativity and strong belief in this project!

Annika Legath and Göran Sunehag for your trust.

Gunilla Kuylenstierna because you made me find my inner child.

Clas von Sydow—you are an amazing human being! Thanks for all the things you've given me, for the knowledge, and for being my friend and mentor.

André Silviera—for your professional skills.

Jonas Sandström because you believed in me, for all the energy and goodwill you have shown us all, and because you believed in your dreams.

I also want to thank Linda Brown, Catarina Falklind-Breschi, Michael Kollberg-Breschi, Mariancila Kim, Yvonne Lin, Anatoli Grigorenko, Kristin Kaspersen, Ann-Sophie

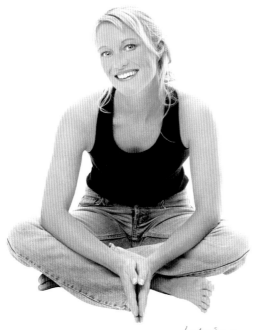

Fjelde, Monika Björn, Bryan and Jan, Sofia Akremi, Sofia Håkonsson, Maria Jacobsson, Alexander Spasojevic, Ari Abromowitz, Jerome Polansky, Mark Polansky, Madeleine Bondesson, Anna Lundin, Susanna Cedric, Jeff Kovatch, the Andersson Family, Carina Boström, Annika Kjellman, Daniel Erneborn, Karin Jensing, Renee Nyberg, Wictoria Höhn, John Sjöberg, Sati Bacchus, and Marianne Zigismond.

Finally a big thank you to Ylab Wellness, Skulpturens hus, Sportguiden, Workouten, N'joy träning och hälse, Aftonbladet, KTH-hallen, and NK Sport och Fritid.

Ulrica

Bibliography

Anodea, Judith. *Eastern body, Western mind.* Celestial Arts. Berkeley, 1996.

Aristotle. *Metaphysics.* The Loeb Classical Library. London, 1956–58.

Beck, Charlotte Joko. *Everyday Zen: Love and Work.* San Francisco, 1989.

Birch, Beryl Bender. *Beyond Poweryoga.* Simon & Schuster. New York, 2000.

Birch, Beryl Bender. *Poweryoga.* Simon & Schuster. New York, 1995.

Bohm, David. *Thought as a System.* Routledge. New York, 1997.

Chopra, Deepak. *Ageless Body, Timeless Mind.* Three Rivers Press. New York, 1994.

Desikachar, T.K.V & Cravens R.H. *Health, Healing and Beyond: Yoga & The Living Tradition of Krishnamacharya.* Aperture Foundation, 1998.

Desikachar, T.K.V. *The Heart of Yoga: Developing a Personal Practice.* Inner Traditions International. Rochester, Vermont, 1995.

Feurstein, Georg & Miller, Jeanine. *The Essence of Yoga.* Inner Traditions, USA, 1998.

Greenfield, Susan. *The Human Brain.* Basic Books. New York, 1997.

Iyengar, B.K.S. *Light on Yoga.* Thorsons Aquarian Press, 1991.

Johari, Harish. *Chakras, Energy Centers of Transformation.* Destinys Books, USA, 1987.

Jois, Sri, K. Pattadhi. *Yoga Mala.* Patanjali Yoga Shala, New York, 1999.

Kaku, Michio & Thompson, Jennifer. *Beyond Einstein.* Doubleday. New York, 1995.

Lalvani, Vimla. *Classic Yoga.* Hamlyn Publishing. London, 1996.

May, Rollo. *The Courage to Create.* Norton, 1994.

Myss, Caroline. *Anatomy of the Spirits.* Three Rivers Press. New York, 1996.

Rahula, Walpola. *What the Buddha Taught.* Grove Press. New York, 1959.

Smith, Houston. *The Illustrated World's Religions: A Guide to Our Wisdom Traditions.* Harpers Publishing. San Francisco, 1991.

Swenson, David. *Ashtanga Yoga—The practice manual.* Ashtanga Yoga Productions. Houston, 1999.

Watts, Alan W. *The Way of Zen.* Thames & Hudson, Penguin Group. New York, 1957.

Patanjali. *Yoga Sutras.* Thorsons Aquarian Press, 1996.

Web sites:

www.poweryoga.com
www.power-yoga.com
www.yrec.com
www.baronbaptiste.com
www.yogajournal.com

Index

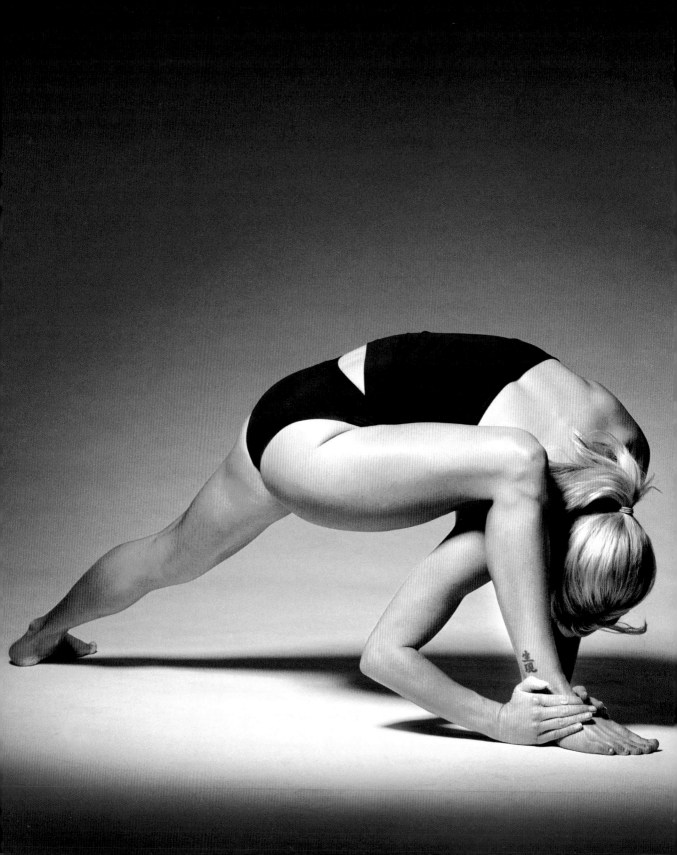